Digital Transformation & Health 4.0

The New (R)evolution

Enrico Guardelli

Copyright © 2024 Enrico Guardelli

All rights reserved

Certain portions of the book may not be reproduced, stored in a retrieval system, or transmitted in any form or by any means, electronic, mechanical, photocopying, recording, or otherwise, without the express written permission of the publisher.

Cover concept by: MedTechBiz

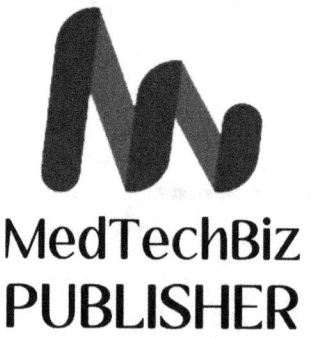

MedTechBiz
PUBLISHER

Table of Contents

Table of Contents..2
Introduction..4
The Digital Revolution in Health 4.0.................................. 7
Digital Health: Concepts, Fundamentals and Challenges............ 17
The "Patient Journey"..26
Digital Health Technologies..41
    Telemedicine... 44
    Medical Devices and Internet of Things (IoT)............................... 47
    Electronic Health Records (EHR)...................................... 50
    Health Apps... 53
    Wearables and Smart Devices.. 55
Training, Education and Organizational Culture......................... 58
Digital Health in Different Contexts.. 63
    Success Stories and Case Studies...69
    Artificial Intelligence in Medicine.. 73
    Big Data... 86
    Blockchain.. 90
    Robotic Surgery... 95
Health Data Protection Laws... 102
    General Data Protection Regulation (GDPR)........................... 110
    Health Insurance Portability and Accountability Act (HIPAA)......114
    General Data Protection Law (LGPD)..................................119
    Personal Data Protection and Electronic Documents Act (PIPEDA)

121
- Privacy Law (Australia).. 124
- Challenges of the LGPD.. 126

Security Measures and Cybersecurity Risks.....................131
Startups and Medtech in Medicine.. 140
Data Interoperability in Healthcare.. 148
Command Center...157
Open Health... 167
Digital Maturity in Healthcare Institutions....................................187
Conclusion... 191
Glossary of Technical Terms.. 194
Bibliographic References... 196
- Books and academic articles... 196
- Magazine and Newspaper Articles.. 202
- Official Reports and Documents.. 203
- Online resources and websites..204
- Conferences and Symposiums.. 207
- Legislation and Regulation... 208

Introduction

In the dynamic and increasingly interconnected healthcare landscape, technology plays a critical role in the transformation and evolution of healthcare.

From the rise of electronic medical records to the development of health tracking apps, digital health has revolutionized the way patients receive care and the way healthcare professionals deliver it.

In this book we explore the complexities and promises of digital health, entering a world where technological innovation and medicine merge to create an exciting future full of possibilities.

As we move forward in this century, we are witnessing an explosion of technological advances that are shaping the way we view health and well-being.

From wearable devices that monitor patients' vital signs to artificial intelligence algorithms that help diagnose diseases early, technology is radically transforming the practice of medicine.

At the same time, the global health context faces unprecedented challenges, such as an aging population, the increase in chronic diseases and the global pandemic.

We explore current and future trends in digital health, examining how technology is applied to improve the quality of care, increase access to medical services, and empower patients to manage their own health.

However, we consider the ethical, regulatory and security challenges that accompany this digital revolution, ensuring that the benefits of technology are achieved in a responsible and inclusive manner.

As we venture into this exciting field of digital health, it is imperative that we consider not only the opportunities it offers, but also the responsibilities it imposes.

This book is a comprehensive exploration of the present and future of digital health, aimed at healthcare professionals, researchers, policymakers, and anyone interested in understanding how technology is shaping the future of healthcare.

Together we explore the limits of innovation and paths to a healthier, more connected future.

The Digital Revolution in Health 4.0

"Health 4.0" represents the next phase in the evolution of the healthcare sector. Driven by the integration of advanced digital technologies, it aims to radically transform healthcare delivery by promoting data interoperability, treatment personalization and a patient-centric approach.

As digital health expert Nosta (2018) states, "Health 4.0 is about the convergence of emerging technologies such as artificial intelligence, genomics, IoT and data analytics to revolutionize the way we manage our health and well-being. ".

In the era of the digital revolution in healthcare, the transformation is profound and continuous, with rapid evolution of information and communication technologies.

This change is reshaping the way healthcare is delivered, improving the efficiency, quality and accessibility of services.

The integration of digital technologies in healthcare has the potential to "empower patients, improve clinical outcomes and reduce costs" - Topol (2012).

Digitization of health data, telemedicine, and remote monitoring devices are just a few of the innovations that are shaping the modern healthcare landscape.

One of the most notable aspects of this revolution is the emergence of electronic health records (EHR), which centralize and digitize patient information, facilitating access and coordination between different healthcare providers.

According to Buntin et al. (2011), EHR adoption can "significantly improve the quality and safety of patient care" by reducing medical errors and ensuring that healthcare professionals have access to the most recent and accurate information.

Telemedicine has also played a crucial role in the digital healthcare revolution, especially during the COVID-19 pandemic, when the need for social distancing accelerated its adoption.

Studies indicate that telemedicine not only improves access to care, but can also be more convenient and efficient for patients and healthcare professionals (Keesara, Jonas, & Schulman, 2020).

Additionally, the development of wearable technologies and remote monitoring devices is allowing patients to better manage their health conditions in real time.

These devices can monitor a variety of parameters such as heart rate, glucose levels and sleep patterns, providing valuable data that can be shared with healthcare professionals for more proactive and personalized care.

The patient-centered approach is one of the greatest promises of the digital revolution in healthcare, as it promotes greater patient autonomy and engagement in their own health journey.

Therefore, the digital revolution in healthcare is fundamentally transforming the way care is delivered and received.

With the continued integration of innovative technologies and increasing emphasis on personalization and efficiency of care, digital health is positioned to offer significant benefits to both patients and healthcare professionals.

As Topol and Buntin (2019) point out, digitalization in healthcare is not just a passing trend, but a necessary evolution that is reshaping the future of medicine.

Paperless solutions involve the digitization of processes, the use of advanced technologies and the implementation of electronic systems that replace physical documents.

This change not only simplifies information management but also improves the quality of patient care and data security.

It is an inevitable evolution, driven by the need to improve operational efficiency, reduce costs and improve the quality of patient care.

One of the main solutions in this context is the adoption of the Electronic Patient Record (PEP), which replaces paper medical records with digital versions accessible to health professionals in real time.

This change not only speeds access to patient information, but also improves diagnostic accuracy and care coordination, resulting in more integrated and effective care.

It is also relevant that electronic prescription of medicines is another key solution in the transition to a paperless environment.

By eliminating the need for paper prescriptions, electronic prescribing significantly reduces medication errors, increases patient safety, and makes it easier for pharmacists and other healthcare professionals to track prescriptions.

This approach also simplifies the prescription renewal process and communication between members of the medical team, promoting more efficient collaboration.

Digitizing intake forms, informed consents, and other administrative documents is another important step in this process. By replacing physical documents with digital versions, healthcare institutions can reduce the time and resources required to process these documents, as well as reduce the need for physical storage space.

It not only streamlines administrative processes, but also contributes to more sustainable and efficient management of the institution's resources.

Online scheduling platforms are becoming increasingly popular and replacing old paper calendars.

They allow patients and healthcare professionals to schedule and manage appointments more efficiently, reducing wait times, minimizing scheduling conflicts, and improving the patient experience.

With easy and convenient access, patients have more control over their appointment schedule, while healthcare professionals can optimize the use of available time and resources.

Another paperless solution is the adoption of electronic billing and coding processes. These automated systems simplify the financial administration of health institutions, reducing errors and accelerating reimbursement for services provided.

With less paperwork and manual processes, organizations can improve financial efficiency and dedicate more resources to direct patient care.

Therefore, the adoption of these solutions promotes greater operational efficiency. Automated and digitized processes are faster, less error-prone and require fewer human resources, resulting in more efficient operations and reduced operating costs.

Cost reduction is another important benefit of paperless solutions. Going paperless reduces costs associated with printing, storing and managing physical documents.

Resources previously dedicated to maintaining physical records can be reallocated to priority areas, such as purchasing modern medical equipment or hiring additional staff.

In summary, paperless solutions in healthcare institutions offer a variety of benefits that improve operational efficiency, reduce costs, improve the quality of patient care, and ensure data security.

These solutions not only modernize healthcare processes, but also contribute to a better and safer experience for patients and healthcare professionals.

One of the main challenges is the significant initial cost associated with the implementation of electronic systems and related technologies. More than investing in software and hardware, there are staff training costs and potential operational disruptions during the implementation process.

Another important challenge is staff training. Introducing new technologies requires employees to become familiar with new systems and processes, which can require a considerable amount of time and resources.

Effective training is essential to ensure employees can use new tools efficiently and productively, minimizing potential errors and maximizing the benefits of paperless solutions.

Systems integration can be complex and requires careful planning to ensure a smooth and seamless transition.

The adoption of paperless solutions is a transformative trend in the healthcare sector, offering significant benefits in terms of efficiency, cost, quality of care and sustainability.

Despite implementation challenges, the potential benefits make this transition a desirable goal for healthcare institutions seeking to modernize their operations and improve patient service.

With strategic planning and investment in training and security, the transition to a paperless environment can be carried out successfully, bringing important advances to the healthcare sector.

Digital Health: Concepts, Fundamentals and Challenges

Digital health can be defined as "the multidisciplinary field of Internet-based and technology-related health information, products and services, ranging from mobile health (mHealth) to electronic health (eHealth) and other emerging disciplines" (Eysenbach, 2001).

This field encompasses other technological innovations such as electronic health records (EHR), telemedicine, wearables, artificial intelligence and big data, among other tools and systems that facilitate health monitoring, diagnosis, treatment and management. remotely and efficiently.

This definition, proposed by Gunther Eysenbach in his article "What is e-health?", highlights the breadth and interdisciplinarity of digital health, emphasizing its connection with technology and its application in different health contexts.

According to Eysenbach (2001), eHealth is a broad term that describes "the application of digital technologies to health, encompassing a wide range of activities and innovations that aim to improve health and healthcare through the use of information technologies." and communication".

mHealth , or mobile health, refers to the use of mobile devices, such as smartphones and tablets, to support medical and public health practice. Applications and technologies designed to monitor health, provide medical information, support self-care, and facilitate communication between patients and healthcare professionals.

From exercise and diet tracking to medication reminders and access to electronic medical records. These mobile tools are becoming increasingly popular due to their convenience, accessibility, and ability to improve patient engagement and health outcomes.

Digital health not only facilitates access to and delivery of healthcare, but also promotes a more patient-centered approach, allowing people to monitor their own health and participate more actively in managing their health conditions.

According to Kay et al. (2001), digital health "empowers patients by providing them with information and tools that enable more effective management of their health and well-being."

Thus, digital health represents a significant transformation in the way healthcare is provided and managed, promoting efficiency, accessibility and personalization of healthcare services through the use of digital technologies.

Although it may seem like a modern phenomenon, digital health has roots that date back to the beginning of the use of communication technologies in medicine. Using the telephone for remote medical consultations and faxing x-rays are some of the first examples.

With the advent of the Internet and personal computers in the 1980s, the first electronic medical record systems and the first attempts at telemedicine emerged.

The introduction of the Internet into everyday life and the expansion of communication networks in the 1990s allowed the development of more sophisticated electronic health record (EHR) systems and the initiation of medical consultations through videoconferencing.

Between the years 2000 - 2009, smartphones became popular and the first health applications (mHealth) emerged in more developed countries. Telemedicine has begun to gain ground, especially in remote areas.

In the 2010s we can highlight advances in wearable devices, such as smart watches with heart rate monitors. Exponential growth of digital health data and beginning of the integration of big data and artificial intelligence in the analysis of this data.

The COVID-19 pandemic has accelerated the adoption of digital health technologies on a global scale in recent years, requiring legal regulation of the activity and emphasizing the importance of remote and technology-based health solutions.

Therefore, we can define "digital health" as an emerging field that integrates information and communication technologies with the practice of medicine and health services.

Digital health terminology also encompasses terms such as interoperability, remote monitoring, IoT (Internet of Things) in healthcare, reflecting the diversity of technologies and approaches that are transforming the way healthcare is delivered and managed.

Understanding these concepts and terminology is essential for healthcare professionals, technology developers, and policymakers as they navigate and shape the future of digital healthcare services.

The introduction of digital technologies in healthcare has had profound impacts, transforming the way healthcare is delivered.

This set of solutions has improved the efficiency and quality of care, allowing for faster and more precise care.

For Topol (2019), the digitalization of health has the potential to empower patients, offering them direct access to their health information and increasing their ability to self-manage chronic diseases.

By providing access to more accurate and up-to-date health data, digital systems help healthcare professionals diagnose and treat diseases. With more complete and accessible information about a patient's medical history, doctors can make more informed decisions and provide more personalized and effective care.

Automating administrative and clinical tasks, such as scheduling appointments, issuing prescriptions, and recording patient data, reduces the time and costs associated with healthcare.

This allows healthcare professionals to spend more time directly caring for patients, improving the overall quality of care.

However, the implementation of these technologies also poses significant challenges. First, the security and privacy of patient data are key concerns.

Protecting sensitive information from unauthorized access and cyberattacks is essential to ensuring patient trust and the integrity of digital health systems.

Another important challenge is the inequality of access to digital technologies. Not all people have equal access to mobile devices, high-speed Internet, or digital skills, creating a digital divide that can widen health disparities.

Interoperability between different health systems continues to be an obstacle that prevents the efficient exchange of information between different platforms.

Kaplan (2016) highlights that it is crucial to develop strong cybersecurity policies and clear regulations to protect patient privacy and ensure data integrity.

These challenges require a collaborative approach between technology developers, healthcare professionals and policymakers to ensure that the benefits of digitalization are fully realized without compromising patient safety and trust.

As technology advances rapidly, it is necessary to develop and implement updated policies and regulations that address issues such as safety standards, legal liability, and patient privacy.

There may be resistance to technology adoption, as many healthcare professionals may resist implementing digital systems due to concerns about the learning curve and changes in clinical practice.

Overcoming these barriers requires a coordinated effort to provide adequate training, technical support, and incentives for technology adoption.

For digital health to be successful, there must be a balance between promoting innovation and protecting the interests of patients and healthcare professionals.

Digital health and the patient journey are intrinsically intertwined, and technology plays a key role in every step of the healthcare process.

From searching for health information to post-treatment follow-up, digital solutions have the potential to improve the patient experience at every stage.

The "Patient Journey"

The "Patient Journey" is a key concept in healthcare and refers to the process a patient goes through from first contact with the healthcare system to the completion of treatment or care.

Gupta et al. (2016) considers the "Patient Journey" to be a holistic representation of the patient's interactions and experiences with health services over time, including everything from seeking initial information about symptoms to performing tests, treatments and post-treatment follow-up.

From the perspective of Smith et al. (2018), the patient journey can be divided into several distinct stages, each with its own challenges and opportunities.

These steps include recognizing the need for medical care, seeking information and guidance, accessing health services, participating in the treatment process, and transitioning to follow-up or post-treatment care.

However, it is important to highlight that the patient journey is not linear and can be influenced by a variety of factors, such as the severity of the health condition, patient preferences, availability of resources, and quality of care services. medical.

As mentioned by Johnson et al. (2020), understanding and mapping the patient journey is essential to identify points of improvement in healthcare service delivery, personalize care to individual patient needs, and ensure a continuous and integrated care experience.

A patient's journey through a healthcare institution involves multiple steps that digitization is transforming in all of their care.

The digital journey begins with recognition and education, when, based on knowledge of the symptoms, information is sought about your health status.

In the digital age, patients rely on a variety of online tools and resources to self-assess and seek initial information about their health.

These resources include self-assessment tools and digital educational resources, which allow users to enter specific symptoms and receive a preliminary analysis, making it easier to understand their health problems before even consulting a health professional.

For example, apps like Ada and WebMD Symptom Checker allow users to enter their symptoms and get a list of possible health conditions.

The apps use advanced algorithms and medical databases to provide preliminary recommendations, helping patients decide whether they should seek immediate medical attention or wait to see if symptoms go away on their own.

Online platforms such as NHS Symptom Checker in the UK offer similar services, allowing patients to describe their symptoms and receive guidance on next steps. They often provide additional information about the severity of symptoms and when to seek emergency help.

In addition to self-assessment tools, digital educational resources play a crucial role in educating patients about their health conditions and available treatment options.

Many doctors and health organizations maintain blogs that offer detailed articles on various health conditions, treatments, and prevention strategies. Written in accessible language, these blogs often answer common patient questions.

Platforms such as YouTube and websites of healthcare organizations such as the Mayo Clinic offer a wide range of educational and explanatory videos on complex medical conditions in a visual and simplified way, making them easier for patients to understand.

The use of visual infographics that combine text and images is also valid to explain medical information in a clear and concise way. They are especially useful for describing biological processes, treatment options, and prevention tips. Organizations like the American Heart Association often use infographics to educate the public about cardiovascular health.

By utilizing these resources, informed patients can begin their healthcare journey with a solid foundation of knowledge, facilitating more productive interactions with healthcare professionals.

Access to and scheduling medical appointments has been significantly transformed by digital health. The possibility of self-scheduling reduces waiting time for appointments and exams, also optimizing administrative processes and medical availability.

Patients often face long wait times for appointments, tests, and procedures, which can delay diagnosis and treatment, worsen the patient's condition, and increase anxiety.

The lack of availability of specialists or convenient appointment times is a recurring problem, making it difficult for patients to obtain timely care, especially in areas with a shortage of healthcare professionals.

These online scheduling platforms allow patients to conveniently book medical appointments through apps or websites, offering a clear view of the availability of different healthcare professionals.

The facility not only speeds up the appointment scheduling process, but also increases transparency, allowing patients to choose times that best suit their needs.

Following the revolution in access to health, teleconsultations and telemedicine offer a practical and efficient alternative, especially beneficial for people with reduced mobility or who live in remote areas.

Telemedicine eliminates the need to travel, reduces wait time, and allows for faster, more effective care.

It was particularly important in times of pandemic such as Covid-19, where the need for social distancing makes in-person consultations less viable. Facilitating the monitoring of chronic diseases provides continuous and regular monitoring.

Innovations in access and scheduling not only benefit patients, but also have a positive impact on the management of healthcare services.

With the digitalization of these processes, better organization of health professionals' schedules is achieved, optimizing the use of available time and resources.

At the same time, digital platforms collect valuable data on service schedules and patterns, which can be analyzed to improve operational efficiency and the quality of services provided.

Another area where technology is having an important impact is in digital diagnosis. Artificial intelligence (AI) and big data analytics are becoming indispensable tools to support clinical diagnosis.

AI tools can analyze large volumes of medical data, including X-ray images, CT scans, and MRIs, to identify patterns and anomalies that may not be easily detectable with the naked eye.

For example, advanced algorithms are able to detect early signs of cancer, heart disease and other serious conditions with great accuracy.

This not only increases the speed and accuracy of diagnoses, but also allows healthcare professionals to make more informed decisions and offer more effective treatments.

These technological innovations are transforming the way diagnoses are made and care is delivered. The integration of digital tools and artificial intelligence in the consultation and diagnosis processes allows for more personalized and proactive medicine.

The ability to analyze data in real time and quickly provide accurate diagnoses can save lives, improve treatment outcomes, and increase the efficiency of healthcare systems.

As technology continues to evolve, the role of teleconsultations and digital diagnosis is expected to become even more central in medical practice, redefining standards of care and driving the quality of healthcare services.

Once the diagnosis is identified, the patient is referred for follow-up and treatment. Digital solutions that use health management applications and remote monitoring devices have contributed to this stage.

Mobile apps, such as MySugr for diabetes and Medisafe for medication reminders, allow patients to manage their chronic illnesses, medications, and medical appointments effectively.

Remote monitoring devices, such as wearables and connected sensors, monitor vital signs and other health metrics in real time. Transmitting data directly to healthcare professionals allows for continuous monitoring and adjustment of treatments as necessary.

Examples include connected blood pressure monitors and continuous glucose sensors, which improve health management and rapid response to changes in patient status.

In parallel, patient support platforms play a crucial role in maintaining health and wellbeing by offering online communities and forums where patients can share their experiences, get support and advice from others with similar conditions.

Thus, these solutions provide a safe and welcoming space, where patients feel understood and less isolated, improving their commitment to medical care and their adherence to prescribed treatments.

Digital wellness programs are another iconic component of ongoing patient support. Online applications and programs, which promote healthy habits such as balanced eating and physical activity, use gamification techniques to keep users motivated.

Continuous monitoring and personalized feedback help patients maintain their health goals, promoting lasting and sustainable behavior change.

In addition to improving physical health, these programs also improve mental well-being by providing a holistic approach to healthcare.

Therefore, digitizing the "Patient Journey" provides important benefits, accessibility being one of the main ones.

Healthcare system efficiency is improved by reducing appointment wait times, simplifying scheduling, and optimizing communication between patients and healthcare professionals.

Another point to highlight is personalization, with digital tools that allow treatments adapted to the individual needs of each patient, considering their medical history and personal preferences.

The lack of clear communication between healthcare professionals and patients is a major problem. Patients may not understand their diagnoses, treatment plans, or care instructions, resulting in noncompliance and errors in self-care.

Care that does not take into account patients' individual needs and preferences decreases patient satisfaction and can negatively affect treatment effectiveness.

Through digital health apps and platforms, patient engagement is increased, encouraging active health management and promoting a healthier lifestyle.

To complete the digital patient journey, continuous monitoring is facilitated by connected devices, enabling real-time monitoring of health conditions, improving clinical outcomes and offering greater peace of mind to patients and healthcare professionals. .

Although digitalization brings numerous benefits, the patient journey is fraught with challenges that can significantly impact the quality of their care and the overall experience at the healthcare institution.

Problems arise at different stages of the process, from admission to discharge and follow-up, and can compromise the effectiveness of the care provided.

From concerns about data security and privacy to issues related to inequality of access and resistance to the adoption of new technologies by healthcare professionals, the challenges of the digital patient journey highlight the need for thoughtful approaches and innovative solutions to ensure a smooth and effective transition. to digital health services.

Ensuring that patient health data is protected from unauthorized access and privacy violations is critical to maintaining patient trust and complying with regulations such as GDPR in Europe and HIPAA in the United States. Implementing strong security measures, such as encryption and access controls, is essential to protect sensitive information and prevent data leaks.

Digital access is a concern that cannot be neglected. Ensuring that all patients, regardless of geographic location or socioeconomic status, have access to digital health technologies can prevent inequalities in care delivery.

Lack of continuity of care, especially when moving from one level of care to another (for example, from hospital to primary care), can lead to gaps in care, lack of adequate follow-up, and an increased risk of readmissions.

Patients may not adhere to the treatment plan, forget follow-up appointments, or not know how to manage their health conditions at home.

Patients often have difficulty accessing their own medical records, making it difficult to track their own treatment and make informed decisions.

Therefore, it is undeniable that the patient's journey in digital health has been transformative in the healthcare experience. Digital technologies can integrate all stages of this journey, significantly improving outcomes by promoting more patient-centered care.

Patient empowerment is essential for true transformation in healthcare. When patients have information about their health, including ongoing monitoring data, they become more involved in their own care, make informed decisions, and engage in healthy behaviors.

More than improving individual health outcomes, it also promotes a more collaborative approach between patients and healthcare professionals, resulting in better overall healthcare system outcomes.

Digital Health Technologies

Digital health technologies play a critical role at every stage of the patient journey, offering quick access to health information, facilitating communication between healthcare professionals, enabling virtual consultations and remote monitoring, and empowering patients to manage their own health in a more active and collaborative way. .

Digital health and the patient journey are intrinsically intertwined, and technology plays a key role in every step of the healthcare process.

For example, mobile applications and online platforms offer quick access to healthcare resources and allow patients to manage their conditions autonomously, allowing them to make informed decisions about their health.

Electronic health record (EHR) and telemedicine systems facilitate communication between patients and healthcare professionals, reducing geographic barriers and improving access to care.

By integrating digital health into the patient journey, it is possible to promote a more patient-centric, personalized and efficient approach that aims to meet individual needs and improve clinical outcomes.

Digital health technologies play a crucial role in every step of the patient journey, providing a more integrated and patient-centric experience.

From searching for health information to post-treatment monitoring, these digital solutions offer significant benefits.

During treatment, electronic health record (EHR) systems facilitate documentation and information sharing between healthcare professionals, ensuring more effective and coordinated communication.

Telemedicine allows virtual consultations and remote monitoring, eliminating geographic barriers and providing greater convenience to patients.

Throughout the journey, digital health technologies enable patients to be more active in managing their own health, promoting a more collaborative and personalized approach to healthcare.

Telemedicine

Telemedicine, according to author Bashshur, Shannon and Krupinski (2019), is defined as "the practice of medicine at a distance, using communication technologies to provide health services, where distance is a barrier to medical assistance."

Bashshur et al. (2016) conceptualize telemedicine to expand access to health services, especially in remote and underserved areas, where the availability of medical professionals and resources is limited.

This allows patients who previously faced geographic or mobility barriers to access specialized care.

According to Whitten et al. (2007), telemedicine can generate significant cost savings for health systems by reducing transportation expenses to medical appointments, unnecessary hospital admissions, and repeat visits to the emergency room.

Telemedicine can be performed in real time (synchronous) or asynchronous, where information is sent and analyzed later.

It is not a new concept. Its roots go back more than half a century. The first documented use of telemedicine was in the 1960s, when NASA began monitoring the health of astronauts in orbit through telemetry systems.

At the same time, the US National Institute of Mental Health used video conferencing to provide psychiatric care to patients in remote locations.

The proliferation of personal computers, the advent of broadband Internet, the popularization of smartphones and other mobile devices have propelled telemedicine to new heights.

Today, telemedicine has become an integral part of modern healthcare systems for several reasons, such as reducing costs associated with in-person visits for both patients and healthcare providers.

Teleconsultation platforms are online systems that facilitate communication between healthcare professionals and patients, for security considerations such as data encryption, user authentication, and regulatory compliance with data protection laws.

In fact, telemedicine is revolutionizing the way healthcare is delivered, making it more accessible, efficient, and personalized.

Medical Devices and Internet of Things (IoT)

For Rajkumar Buyya (2018), professor of Computer Science at the University of Melbourne, "the Internet of Things (IoT) is a distributed systems architecture that allows remote monitoring and control of physical objects, obtaining feedback in real time. and allowing autonomous decision-making."

Atzori et al. (2010) defines it as "a global infrastructure for the information society, which enables advanced interactive services through the interconnection of physical and virtual objects based on information and communication technologies."

These definitions highlight the ability of IoT devices to interact with each other and the environment, creating an interconnected system that enables automation and real-time data analysis.

As for Gubbi et al. (2013), IoT devices have the potential to offer a variety of benefits, including task automation, remote monitoring, real-time data collection, and intelligent decision making. These benefits can be applied to various sectors, such as health, agriculture, transportation and manufacturing, among others.

The McKinsey Global Institute report (2015) highlights that IoT can generate significant economic impact, estimated at trillions of dollars by 2025, through greater operational efficiency, the creation of new business models and improvements in quality of life.

The use of IoT devices can reduce medical costs and improve the operational efficiency of health systems by providing real-time data to healthcare professionals, facilitating faster and more accurate interventions.

It can measure vital signs such as heart rate, activity levels, sleep, and oxygen saturation. Remote sensors can be used at home to monitor blood pressure, blood glucose levels and weight.

What's more, these devices promote treatment personalization as the data collected helps create care plans tailored to each patient's individual needs, resulting in better health outcomes and greater patient satisfaction.

Connected medical devices have strategic importance as an enabling technology for digital transformation in various sectors of the economy.

Electronic Health Records (EHR)

Electronic health records (EHR) are patient medical records in digital format that can be shared between healthcare providers, hospitals, and patients.

The implementation and use of EHRs has transformed the way health data is managed and used, providing numerous benefits to healthcare professionals and patients.

Blumenthal (2011) cites that "EHRs are critical tools for improving the quality, safety, and efficiency of healthcare." The implementation of these systems allows health information to be consolidated in a single accessible place, facilitating the exchange of information between different health professionals and institutions.

When implemented, there is an improvement in care coordination, reductions in redundancy of tests and procedures, and improvements in the accuracy of diagnoses and treatments.

EHRs can incorporate alerts and reminders to help healthcare providers adhere to clinical guidelines and better manage patients' chronic conditions.

The implementation of Electronic Health Records (EHR) has a significant impact on care coordination and the quality of care provided to patients.

As long as they are interoperable, EHRs can exchange information between different health professionals and institutions, allowing a complete and integrated view of the patient's medical history. This ensures that everyone involved in a patient's care has access to the most up-to-date and relevant information, promoting better coordination of care.

According to Bates et al. (2003), "EHRs improve the quality of care by facilitating communication between healthcare providers and providing easier and faster access to clinical information."

The ability to quickly access patient data allows healthcare professionals to make informed and timely decisions, reducing the incidence of medical errors.

Health Apps

Health and fitness apps are digital tools designed to help people manage their health and well-being. These apps offer a wide range of features, from fitness tracking and diet tracking to medication reminders and health data tracking.

According to Patel et al. (2015), health and fitness applications are defined as "mobile applications that aim to improve the health and well-being of their users through various functionalities, such as physical activity tracking, diet tracking, "monitoring sleep patterns and providing health information."

The tool has the potential to offer a number of benefits to users. First, they provide greater awareness of health habits and encourage positive behavioral changes.

By providing instant feedback on progress toward health goals, these apps can motivate users to adopt healthier, more active lifestyles.

Therefore, health apps make it easier to track and manage personal health. Users can track metrics such as heart rate, calories burned, sleep patterns, and food intake, gaining valuable insights into their health and behavior.

Because data can be shared with healthcare professionals for personalized assessment and guidance, it facilitates a more proactive and preventative approach to healthcare.

With the increasing availability of mobile devices and connectivity, these apps have become a powerful tool to empower people to take a more active role in their own health and well-being.

Thus, health applications represent an important facet of the digital revolution in health, offering resources and support to promote healthy lifestyles and improve quality of life.

Wearables and Smart Devices

Wearables and smart devices refer to technological equipment that can be worn on the body and that have the ability to monitor, record and transmit data related to the user's health and well-being.

These devices include smartwatches, fitness bracelets, heart rate monitors, and even smart clothing that can measure various health metrics.

For Patel and Wang (2020), "wearables are electronic devices that consumers can wear and that allow them to collect data about their physical activities and health parameters, often in real time."

These devices are equipped with sensors that collect physiological data, such as heart rate, activity levels, sleep quality, among others.

Wearable and smart devices bring a number of benefits to both individual users and the healthcare system as a whole.

Firstly, they allow for continuous health monitoring, providing real-time data that can be used to detect any abnormalities or health problems early.

According to Jackson and Boren (2019), "Wearable devices offer an unprecedented opportunity for continuous health monitoring, enabling rapid and personalized interventions."

More than anything, these devices encourage a healthier lifestyle by providing constant, motivating information about the user's physical activity and health habits.

Another important benefit is the ability of these devices to integrate with digital health platforms, allowing the data collected to be shared with healthcare professionals. You will be able to improve the management of chronic diseases and personalize treatments based on precise and detailed data.

Analysis of this data can lead to deeper insights into patient health and the effectiveness of treatments, promoting more personalized and preventive medicine.

Continuous health monitoring, enabled by digital technologies, offers a real-time view of an individual's health status, enabling early and personalized interventions.

This practice allows us to detect patterns, trends and anomalies that may not be evident in specific medical consultations, facilitating prevention, early diagnosis and management of health conditions.

Therefore, continuous monitoring can promote greater awareness of lifestyle and habits that impact health, empowering people to take proactive steps to improve their overall well-being.

Training, Education and Organizational Culture

The transition to digital health requires a significant focus on training and education to ensure that healthcare professionals are prepared to use new technologies and systems effectively.

Taken together, creating an organizational culture that supports innovation and adaptation is crucial to the success of digital transformation in healthcare.

Digital health training involves training healthcare professionals in the use of technologies such as EHRs, telemedicine systems, and other digital tools.

From the point of view of Gagnon et al. (2012), "continuing training and professional development are essential for health professionals to acquire the skills necessary to use health information technologies effectively."

This training not only improves the technical competence of professionals, but also increases their confidence and acceptance of new technologies.

Creating an organizational culture that encourages innovation is critical to the successful implementation of digital health. Westphal et al. (2010) highlight that "an organizational culture that values continuous learning and innovation facilitates the adoption of new technologies and practices."

In any case, it promotes a mindset open to change, encouraging interdepartmental collaboration and supporting leadership in digital health.

The combined impact of proper training and a supportive organizational culture can lead to significant improvements in operational efficiency, quality of care, and patient satisfaction.

Well-trained professionals and an adaptable organization are better equipped to meet the challenges and seize the opportunities presented by the digitalization of healthcare.

Educating patients about the use of health technologies is essential to maximize the benefits of these tools and promote greater autonomy and involvement in managing their own health.

As the healthcare industry digitizes, patients are increasingly encouraged to use technologies such as patient portals, mobile health apps, and remote monitoring devices.

Gee et al. (2015) emphasize that "educating patients about the use of health technologies can significantly increase patient engagement and improve health outcomes."

Lack of knowledge or confidence in the use of these technologies can be a significant barrier to their adoption.

Therefore, providing clear instructions, training, and ongoing support is critical to ensuring patients feel comfortable and able to use these tools effectively.

Patient education methods may include online tutorials, in-person workshops, printed materials, and technical support. It is important to adapt educational material to the needs and abilities of patients, taking into account factors such as age, health knowledge, and familiarity with technology.

For example, video tutorials and step-by-step guides can be especially helpful for patients who are new to using digital technologies.

Effectively educating patients about the use of technologies can lead to a number of benefits, including better management of chronic diseases, greater adherence to treatment, and more efficient communication with healthcare professionals.

Well-informed and empowered patients are more likely to use these technologies continuously and effectively, which can result in better overall health and reduced long-term healthcare costs.

From the perspective of O'Donoghue et al. (2019), "digital health policies should be developed taking into account patient needs, integration with existing health systems, and best practices in terms of data security and privacy."

As such, policymakers and regulators must work closely with healthcare professionals, technology companies, and patients to develop clear and comprehensive guidelines to ensure the ethical and effective use of digital technologies in healthcare. .

What's more, digital health regulation also plays an important role in promoting interoperability between health information systems, enabling the secure and efficient exchange of data between different providers and health systems.

Digital Health in Different Contexts

In the clinical context, digital health enables the use of electronic health record (EHR) systems, telemedicine, and remote monitoring tools to facilitate early diagnosis, personalized treatment, and continuous patient monitoring.

These technologies allow healthcare professionals to provide more efficient and accessible care, especially in remote or low-resource areas.

In the hospital environment, digital health manifests itself through integrated hospital management systems, connected medical devices, and robot-assisted surgeries.

These solutions aim to improve operational efficiency, reduce medical errors, and ensure a safer and more comfortable experience for patients during their hospital stay.

At the population level, digital health is used in epidemiological surveillance programs, disease monitoring, public health campaigns and promotion of healthy lifestyles.

Information and communication technologies enable the collection, analysis and dissemination of health data in real time, facilitating evidence-based decision making and the implementation of effective interventions.

Digital health plays a fundamental role in the education and training of healthcare professionals, clinical research and the development of new therapies and treatments.

The use of virtual simulations, augmented reality and artificial intelligence is transforming the way healthcare professionals are trained and how medical research is conducted, accelerating innovation and advancement in medicine.

In summary, digital health encompasses a wide range of applications and contexts, all with the common goal of improving people's health and well-being through technological innovation and the integration of data and health information.

In urban settings, digital health plays a key role in addressing specific challenges associated with population density and the complexity of health systems.

One of the main applications is telemedicine, which allows access to remote health services, reducing the need to physically travel to medical appointments. In fact, it is especially important in urban areas, where traffic and distance can represent significant barriers to accessing healthcare.

Another important application of digital health in urban environments is the analysis of large-scale health data to identify public health trends and patterns.

These analyzes can help health authorities prioritize resources and interventions, predict disease outbreaks, and implement more effective prevention strategies.

In rural settings, digital health plays a crucial role in overcoming geographic and access barriers to healthcare. A key application is telemedicine, which connects patients in remote areas with healthcare experts in urban centers through virtual communication technologies.

Consequently, it significantly reduces the need for long and expensive trips to medical appointments, making healthcare services more accessible and convenient for rural communities.

In addition to telemedicine, mobile health units are another important application of digital health in rural settings.

These vehicles are equipped with advanced medical technologies, such as portable diagnostic devices and mobile Internet connections, allowing healthcare professionals to perform examinations, diagnoses and consultations directly in rural communities.

It is considered especially beneficial in areas where healthcare infrastructure is scarce or non-existent, providing access to quality healthcare where none previously existed.

Additionally, digital health education and training programs are essential to train health professionals in rural areas to effectively use digital technologies. For example, training on how to use health apps, remote monitoring devices, and telemedicine platforms.

By providing these skills, rural health professionals can provide more comprehensive and efficient care to their communities, improving health outcomes and reducing disparities in access to health care.

In developed countries, digital health is characterized by the intensive use of advanced technologies to improve healthcare. The use of artificial intelligence for diagnosis and treatment is considered, leveraging advanced algorithms to interpret medical images and analyze large clinical data sets.

In developing countries, digital health focuses on low-cost, high-efficiency solutions to overcome the challenges of limited infrastructure and resources.

Covers the implementation of disease management mobile applications that provide guidance and support to patients, as well as facilitating access to health information and medical services.

SMS messaging programs are another common tool for disseminating health education and medication reminders in communities with limited Internet access.

Additionally, telemedicine is widely used in remote areas without access to specialists, connecting patients with healthcare professionals through virtual consultations, helping to improve access and quality of healthcare in underserved regions.

Success Stories and Case Studies

Digital health success stories and case studies highlight concrete examples of how technologies are being successfully applied to improve healthcare delivery and patient outcomes.

A notable example is the case study "Reducing Hospital Readmissions Using Telemedicine" by Smith et al. (2019), which demonstrated how the implementation of telemedicine programs for remote patient monitoring after discharge significantly reduced hospital readmission rates and improved continuity of care.

Another relevant case study is the "Use of artificial intelligence for skin cancer screening" conducted by Johnson et al. (2020), which showed how artificial intelligence algorithms can be trained to identify lesions suspicious for skin cancer with high precision, allowing for more efficient and faster detection and facilitating access to early diagnoses and timely treatments.

Furthermore, the success story of "Implementation of electronic medical records in a primary care clinic" described by García et al. (2018), highlighted the benefits of transitioning from paper records to electronic records, including greater accuracy of documentation, coordination of care, and faster access to relevant clinical information.

These case studies illustrate the transformative potential of digital health and provide valuable insights into best practices, challenges and opportunities associated with implementing information and communications technologies in different healthcare contexts.

Emerging Trends and Innovations in the Healthcare Sector

Emerging trends and innovations in healthcare are rapidly shaping the industry landscape, driving significant advances in healthcare delivery and promoting patient well-being.

With the advancement of technology and the convergence of multiple disciplines, we are witnessing an era of unprecedented transformation in the way health is understood, treated and managed.

From artificial intelligence and big data solutions to the wearable revolution and telemedicine, these innovations are redefining the boundaries of what is possible in healthcare.

In this dynamic and exciting context, it is essential to explore the latest trends and discoveries to understand how they are shaping the future of medicine and to prepare for the challenges and opportunities that arise in this constantly evolving environment.

Digital Transformation and Health 4.0 - The New (R)evolution

Artificial Intelligence in Medicine

Artificial intelligence (AI) is an area of computing that focuses on developing systems capable of performing tasks that normally require human intelligence.

John McCarthy, one of the pioneers of AI, defines "artificial intelligence is the science and engineering of producing intelligent machines." These machines are capable of learning from data, solving problems, recognizing patterns and making decisions based on algorithms. In other words, AI allows computers to act intelligently, imitating some human capabilities.

AI involves the use of algorithms and computer systems to perform tasks that typically require human intelligence, such as learning, reasoning, pattern recognition, and decision making. In medicine, AI is becoming a crucial tool to improve the accuracy of diagnoses, personalize treatments and increase the efficiency of healthcare systems.

The application of artificial intelligence in diagnostic imaging has revolutionized medicine by allowing more precise and efficient analysis of radiological examinations.

For example, deep learning algorithms are trained on large data sets to recognize subtle patterns that could indicate the presence of diseases.

These systems can identify abnormalities in X-ray images, MRIs, and CT scans with accuracy comparable to or even greater than that of human radiologists.

This ability to quickly and accurately identify medical conditions has a significant impact on clinical practice, allowing for earlier diagnoses and more effective treatments.

In cases of cancer, for example, early detection can increase the chances of successful treatment and improve outcomes for patients. AI can therefore help radiologists prioritize exams, identifying urgent cases that require immediate attention.

However, despite its benefits, implementing AI in diagnostic imaging also presents challenges. It is necessary to ensure the quality of the data used to train the algorithms, as well as continually validate the performance of the systems in real-world conditions.

It is important to integrate these AI tools seamlessly into clinical workflow, ensuring that radiologists can take full advantage of their potential in daily practice.

Hospitals around the world are adopting artificial intelligence systems to improve diagnostic imaging and improve the efficiency of radiology services. For example, Mount Sinai Hospital in New York implemented an artificial intelligence system to help radiologists detect abnormalities in mammography images, increase accuracy and speed up the patient triage process.

Similarly, St. Joseph's Hospital in London uses artificial intelligence algorithms to analyze CT scans and identify signs of conditions such as pulmonary embolism, speeding up the diagnosis and treatment of critically ill patients.

Another notable example is Heidelberg University Hospital in Germany, which implemented an artificial intelligence system to analyze brain MRI images and aid in the diagnosis of neurodegenerative diseases such as Alzheimer's and Parkinson's.

This system allows for early detection of these conditions, allowing for more effective therapeutic interventions and improving the quality of life of patients.

In the US, Boston Hospital in the United States adopted AI to optimize the scheduling of imaging exams, using predictive algorithms to estimate wait time and equipment availability, ensuring more efficient distribution of resources and reducing patient waiting time.

Siemens Healthineers, one of the world's leading medical technology companies, has developed several artificial intelligence solutions for use in hospitals. One example is the AI-Rad Companion Chest CT software, which uses artificial intelligence algorithms to analyze chest CT scans.

It can automatically identify anatomical structures and disease patterns, helping radiologists interpret images more efficiently and accurately. This Siemens solution improves the productivity of healthcare professionals and accelerates the patient diagnosis process.

GE Healthcare is known for its innovative artificial intelligence solutions in medicine. One example is ViosWorks, a cardiac MRI software that uses artificial intelligence to produce detailed images and 3D reconstructions of the heart in a single exam, saving time and resources.

Another example is Critical Care Suite, an artificial intelligence application that helps with early detection of critical conditions on chest x-rays, such as pneumothorax, streamlining the diagnostic process and improving outcomes for patients.

These GE solutions demonstrate how AI is transforming medicine by delivering faster, more accurate diagnoses.

Philips is also at the forefront of integrating AI into medicine. IntelliSpace Discovery is a data analytics platform that uses AI to help researchers identify patterns and insights in large clinical and imaging data sets.

Its solutions such as IntelliSpace AI Workflow Suite, which uses AI to automate administrative tasks and improve operational efficiency in hospitals.

Virtual assistants and chatbots have become increasingly common tools in the healthcare sector and offer a number of benefits for both healthcare professionals and patients.

Based on AI, they can be used to schedule appointments, detect symptoms, provide information about medications and health conditions, as well as provide emotional and educational support to patients.

Virtual assistants and chatbots can help reduce the workload of healthcare professionals by directing simple queries to automated systems, allowing doctors to focus on more complex cases and provide high-quality care.

A notable example of a virtual assistant in healthcare is "Ask Mayo Clinic," developed by Mayo Clinic. This virtual assistant provides answers to questions about symptoms, diseases, treatments and medications, offering reliable information based on clinical evidence.

Another example is "Babylon Health," a chatbot that allows users to query symptoms, receive personalized health advice, and even schedule remote medical appointments, making healthcare more accessible and convenient.

Personalized medicine is revolutionized by artificial intelligence (AI), which has the ability to analyze vast sets of genomic and clinical data to identify patterns and predict which treatments will be most effective for specific individuals.

By analyzing this data, AI can offer valuable insights into a patient's response to certain medications, allowing for a more precise and personalized approach to treating the disease.

The ability to personalize not only increases the chances of successful treatments, but also reduces side effects, providing a safer and more effective care experience for patients.

A concrete example of this application of AI in personalized medicine is the analysis of genomic data to identify specific mutations related to certain medical conditions.

Based on this information, doctors can select targeted therapies that are most effective for each patient's genetic profile, maximizing positive treatment outcomes.

AI can also help identify biomarkers that indicate disease progression or response to treatment, allowing for more precise and timely adjustments to the therapeutic plan.

This combination of genomic data and predictive analytics is redefining healthcare standards, making personalized medicine an increasingly accessible and effective reality.

Mount Sinai Hospital in New York uses AI to analyze patients' genomic data and develop personalized therapies for diseases such as cancer and cardiovascular disease. Using each patient's genetic information, doctors can prescribe more specific treatments, increasing success rates and minimizing side effects.

Companies like Tempus and Foundation Medicine are examples of organizations operating in the personalized medicine segment with the help of artificial intelligence. Tempus, founded by Eric Lefkofsky, uses clinical and genomic data analysis to develop personalized cancer therapies, helping doctors make more informed treatment decisions.

Additionally, Foundation Medicine, acquired by Roche, specializes in genomic sequencing of tumors and provides detailed information on the genetic characteristics of cancers, guiding doctors in choosing the most effective therapies for patients.

Disease prediction and epidemic management have benefited significantly from the use of artificial intelligence (AI) models.

The models are capable of analyzing a wide range of data, including health records, travel patterns, demographic information and weather data, to identify potential disease outbreaks.

For example, AI algorithms can quickly track and analyze symptom data reported on social media and health platforms to identify geographic areas where cases of a given disease are increasing, allowing for a more agile response by authorities. public health authorities.

AI models can predict the spread of diseases based on transmission patterns and population characteristics.

By analyzing this data in real time, AI systems can provide estimates on the spread of diseases and the likelihood of outbreaks in different regions.

In this sense, public health authorities can implement preventive measures, such as targeted vaccination campaigns and travel restrictions, to contain the spread of diseases and reduce the impact of epidemics and pandemics.

In summary, AI models play a crucial role in disease prediction and epidemic management, providing valuable information for public health decision-making and helping to protect population health.

We can mention BlueDot as a use case for artificial intelligence in disease prediction and epidemic management. Its developed epidemiological surveillance system uses artificial intelligence algorithms to analyze data from multiple sources, such as public health reports, flight data, social media and online news, to detect patterns and identify potential disease outbreaks around the world.

In January 2020, the BlueDot system was one of the first to warn about the spread of the new coronavirus, identifying areas at risk of spread even before health authorities made their alerts official.

In the field of surgical robotics, artificial intelligence is revolutionizing the way surgical procedures are performed with greater millimeter precision and better outcomes for patients.

Leading companies in this segment, such as Intuitive Surgical with its da Vinci system, are at the forefront of this innovation.

The da Vinci system combines robotic precision with surgeon guidance, enabling less invasive procedures in areas such as cardiac, urological, gynecological and gastrointestinal surgery.

The system's ability to perform delicate and complex movements with greater precision has led to shorter recovery times and fewer postoperative complications, significantly improving the patient experience.

As for Intuitive Surgical, other companies are also investing in AI-assisted surgical robotics technologies.

Medtronic, for example, developed the Hugo system, which combines advanced artificial intelligence with cutting-edge robotics to provide exceptional precision and control to surgeons.

This system is designed for a wide range of surgical procedures, from abdominal and thoracic surgeries to procedures in areas such as orthopedics and neurology.

Big Data

Big Data in healthcare is redefining the way data is explored and applied in the medical field, opening new perspectives for healthcare delivery.

As highlighted by Meyer et al. (2018), Big Data's ability to handle massive volumes of information from multiple sources is critical to extracting valuable information that can significantly improve healthcare services.

It is an emerging technology that is profoundly transforming the way data is used in the medical field.

When handling massive volumes of information from diverse sources, such as patient records, genomic data, test results, and connected medical devices, Big Data offers the ability to extract valuable information that can significantly improve healthcare delivery.

This technological revolution has the potential to drive significant advances in areas such as early diagnosis, personalized treatment and disease prevention.

One of the distinctive characteristics of Big Data in healthcare, as highlighted by Housman and Dredze (2015), is its ability to process data quickly and efficiently.

With advanced algorithms and scalable computing power, analysis of large data sets can be performed in real time, enabling the detection of patterns and trends relevant to clinical decision making.

One of the main characteristics of Big Data in the healthcare field is its ability to process data quickly and efficiently. With advanced algorithms and scalable computing power, analysis of large data sets can be performed in real time, enabling the detection of patterns and trends relevant to patient care.

This is especially crucial in situations where quick decisions are needed, such as in cases of medical emergencies or epidemics.

More than speed, Big Data in health is capable of handling a variety of data, as highlighted by Kocaballi et al. (2019). Health data can come in different formats, including text, images, audio and video, and Big Data is capable of integrating and analyzing this heterogeneous information in a cohesive manner.

Therefore, it allows for a more comprehensive understanding of patients' health conditions and more informed decision-making by healthcare professionals.

Identifying individual patterns and predicting potential health complications in advance allows for more proactive and personalized treatment approaches, which can significantly improve clinical outcomes and reduce costs associated with healthcare.

Digital twins, a real-time virtual representation of a physical object or process, are emerging as a powerful tool in the field of Big Data in the healthcare field.

These digital models can capture detailed information about a patient's physiology, genetics, and medical history, offering an accurate and dynamic representation of their health.

By integrating digital twins into Big Data systems, healthcare professionals can perform more accurate simulations and predictive analysis, identifying patterns and correlations that may not be obvious in traditional data.

This allows for a more personalized and preventive approach to patient care, with early interventions based on predictive insights.

Blockchain

Blockchain in healthcare refers to the application of blockchain technology in the healthcare sector, offering an innovative approach to data management and information security.

According to the definition of Halamka et al. (2017), blockchain is a "distributed ledger technology that enables the creation of a shared, immutable digital record of transactions."

Therefore, the information recorded in a blockchain is stored in a decentralized computer network, which increases transparency and security, since each transaction is validated and recorded by consensus between network participants.

Krawiec (2018) highlights that blockchain in healthcare offers the promise of "ensuring the integrity and security of healthcare data, as well as improving interoperability between healthcare systems."

It is especially important in an environment where the exchange of health information between different systems and organizations often faces security and reliability challenges.

The use of blockchain can help mitigate these challenges by providing a secure, immutable record of all healthcare data transactions, from the moment they are created to their final use.

This greater transparency and security can generate greater trust in health information and better collaboration between the different actors in the health system.

Distributed ledger technology has gained importance in recent years due to its ability to provide transparency, security, and decentralization in various applications, including healthcare.

Made up of a network of computers (nodes) that maintain an identical copy of a transaction record, known as a "block", each new block contains a list of valid transactions and is connected to the previous block, forming a chain of blocks.

Once recorded in a block, a transaction is immutable and cannot be changed without the consensus of the majority of network participants.

In the healthcare sector, blockchain offers revolutionary potential for medical data management. Digital medical records can be stored securely and decentralized, allowing patients and healthcare professionals to access and share information efficiently and securely.

In fact, blockchain technology can be used to trace the history of medicines from manufacturing to distribution, guaranteeing their authenticity and reducing the risks of counterfeiting or adulteration.

Medical devices connected to the Internet of Things (IoT) can also be registered and authenticated on the blockchain, ensuring the integrity and security of the data collected.

Additionally, blockchain can be a solution to manage patient consent to share health data, respecting their individual preferences.

Finally, blockchain technology facilitates the secure exchange of research data between institutions, promoting transparency and integrity in the results obtained.

Despite its numerous benefits, blockchain faces significant challenges in the healthcare sector. Scalability, regulation, interoperability, and privacy are important considerations that must be addressed.

However, with a clear understanding of the challenges and benefits, blockchain has the potential to revolutionize the way healthcare data is managed, delivering important benefits for patients, healthcare professionals and sector institutions.

Blockchain has the potential to transform the way healthcare data is managed, shared and protected. With security, transparency, and efficiency, blockchain can promote better collaboration among healthcare stakeholders, thereby improving the quality of care and driving innovation in healthcare.

Although challenges such as scalability, regulation and interoperability need to be overcome so that blockchain can reach its full potential in healthcare.

Robotic Surgery

Robotic surgery in medicine is an advanced approach that combines robotic technology with surgical techniques to perform procedures in a precise and controlled manner.

According to Shah, Amin and Gopal (2021), it involves the use of robotic systems controlled by surgeons to perform interventions with greater precision and dexterity than would be possible with human hands alone.

This technology offers a wide range of applications in various surgical specialties, from cardiac and urological surgeries to gynecological and gastrointestinal procedures.

According to Gagner and Dubuc (2018), robotic surgery is characterized by the use of a robotic platform composed of articulated arms and miniaturized surgical instruments.

The robotic arms are controlled by the surgeon through a command console, which transmits the precise movements of the surgeon's hands to instruments inside the patient's body.

Therefore, it allows for more delicate and precise manipulation of tissues during surgery, resulting in smaller incisions, less damage to surrounding tissues, and a faster recovery for the patient.

Surgical robotics offer a number of advantages compared to traditional methods, including greater precision, shorter hospital stays, less blood loss during surgery, and a lower risk of postoperative complications.

The high-definition visualization provided by robotic systems allows the surgeon a magnified and detailed view of the surgical field, facilitating the identification and removal of diseased tissue with greater precision.

Automation is also driving significant advances in telehealth, allowing surgeons to perform procedures remotely with the help of remotely controlled robotic systems.

Therefore, it can facilitate access to specialized surgical care in remote or underserved areas, as well as enable collaboration between surgeons in different geographic locations.

In other words, robotic surgery represents an important evolution in surgical practice, offering a unique combination of precision, control and accessibility that benefits both patients and healthcare professionals.

The trend is for artificial intelligence to achieve significant advances in terms of efficiency and safety of procedures.

For Wang et al. (2019), AI in robotic surgery refers to the ability of robotic systems to learn from data, recognize patterns, and make autonomous decisions during operations. This capability is essential to improve the precision of the robot's movements and improve assistance to the surgeon.

The application of AI in robotic surgery covers several areas, from preoperative planning to procedure execution.

In planning, AI algorithms can analyze medical images, such as CT scans and MRIs, to help identify anatomical structures and define the best surgical strategy (Patel et al., 2020).

During surgery, AI systems can continuously monitor patient data such as vital signs and physiological parameters, alerting the surgeon to any changes that require immediate intervention.

In fact, AI in robotic surgery also drives innovation in the development of new surgical techniques and procedures. As highlighted by Smith et al. (2021), the ability of AI to process large volumes of data and perform complex analysis allows the development of personalized surgical approaches adapted to the specific needs of each patient.

In this context, the use of machine learning algorithms stands out to optimize the trajectory of surgical instruments, minimizing trauma to surrounding tissues and accelerating postoperative recovery.

Finally, as highlighted by Jones et al. (2018), the integration of AI into robotic surgery represents a significant advance in medicine, providing a powerful combination of robotic precision and artificial intelligence.

This combination promises to revolutionize surgical practice, offering more predictable results, reducing procedure time and improving clinical outcomes for patients.

Augmented Reality (AR) and Virtual Reality (VR)

Augmented Reality (AR) and Virtual Reality (VR) are revolutionizing the way medicine is practiced, offering a range of applications from training healthcare professionals to surgical planning and patient rehabilitation.

AR combines virtual elements with the real environment, while VR creates a completely virtual environment. Both technologies offer important benefits for healthcare.

According to Dr. Rafael Grossmann, a pioneer in the use of Augmented Reality in surgeries, these technologies "have the potential to transform the way doctors practice and patients experience medicine."

Benefits include more immersive and realistic training for healthcare professionals, allowing them to practice complex procedures in a simulated environment before performing them on real patients.

Additionally, AR and VR facilitate preoperative planning by allowing surgeons to view organs and anatomical structures in 3D, which can improve the precision and outcomes of surgeries.

For patients, these technologies can be used in rehabilitation, providing interactive virtual environments that encourage movement and active participation in recovery. As technology advances, AR and VR are expected to become increasingly accessible and integrated into clinical practice, offering exciting new possibilities for future medicine.

Health Data Protection Laws

General health data protection laws are essential to ensure the privacy and security of patients' personal information in the context of health services.

These laws establish guidelines and regulations for the use, storage and sharing of health data, with the goal of protecting people's rights and privacy.

According to Kumar and Puraswani (2020), health data protection laws are defined as "a set of legal rules governing the collection, processing, storage and sharing of health information, with the aim of protecting privacy and confidentiality of patient data.

For Greenberg (2021), "data protection is essential to maintain the integrity and confidentiality of health information, preventing possible violations that could have serious consequences for affected people."

Without a strong legal framework, personal health information can be exposed to risks, from fraud to discrimination.

One of the main foundations of these laws is informed consent. Patients must be adequately informed about how their health data will be collected, used and shared, and must give explicit consent to these practices.

Informed consent is essential to ensure that patients have control over their information and can make informed decisions about their privacy.

As D'Amour and Feizi (2018) state, "informed consent is a fundamental ethical principle that underpins health data protection laws, ensuring that patients have autonomy and control over their personal information."

The need for data security and confidentiality is also among the principles, including measures to protect data against unauthorized access, misuse, loss or breach.

Healthcare organizations must implement appropriate security controls, such as encryption, user authentication, and access audits, to ensure the integrity and confidentiality of patient data.

Highlighted by Li et al. (2019), "data security is an essential component of healthcare data protection laws, ensuring that patients' personal information is protected from cybersecurity threats and other vulnerabilities."

Another guideline is data anonymization, which is the process by which personal information is modified or removed from data sets so that the individuals to whom the data relate can no longer be identified.

By Machanavajjhala et al. (2007), data anonymization is defined as "the process of modifying data to remove or obscure information that could identify specific individuals, so that the data becomes irreversibly anonymous."

This process involves techniques such as removing direct identifiers, such as names and identification numbers, and applying statistical methods to mask individual characteristics of the data, ensuring that people's identities remain protected.

Data anonymization is essential to ensure the privacy and security of personal information, especially in contexts where data will be shared or used for research, analysis or other secondary purposes.

Pseudonymization is defined by Machanavajjhala et al. (2007), pseudonymization is "the replacement of direct identifiers of a record with fictitious identifiers, so that records can be linked to each other without revealing the identity of the individuals."

This technique allows data to continue to be used effectively for legitimate purposes, such as research and analysis, while protecting individuals' identities and minimizing the risk of privacy breaches.

Pseudonymization is often used in conjunction with other data protection measures, such as encryption, to ensure the security and privacy of personal information.

The global context of health data protection varies significantly, reflecting the different approaches and priorities of different countries.

In the United States, the Health Insurance Portability and Accountability Act (HIPAA) sets standards to protect the privacy of medical information, while in the European Union, the General Data Protection Regulation (GDPR) provides a comprehensive approach to data protection, including health data. .

According to Johnson (2020), "the diversity of data protection regulations around the world reflects the complexity and importance of protecting health information in different cultural and legal contexts."

Historically, the evolution of data protection laws in healthcare began to gain steam in the late 20th century as digitization of medical records became more common.

In the United States, HIPAA was enacted in 1996, marking a turning point in the protection of health information. The law establishes security and privacy standards to protect patients' medical data.

In the European Union, the GDPR, which came into force in 2018, replaced the old Data Protection Directive of 1995, expanding individuals' rights over their personal data and imposing stricter obligations on organizations.

Today, with the increasing digitalization of healthcare services and the increased use of technologies such as big data and artificial intelligence, the importance of data protection laws in healthcare is even more evident.

Protecting health data not only prevents privacy breaches, but also ensures that technological innovations are developed and implemented ethically and safely.

Greenberg (2021) highlights that "compliance with data protection laws is crucial to ensuring that emerging technologies in healthcare are adopted in a way that respects patient rights and privacy."

The challenges of implementing and maintaining effective healthcare data protection laws include rapid technological developments, which can outpace existing legislation, and the need to harmonize global regulations.

Johnson (2020) suggests that "one of the biggest challenges is ensuring that laws are flexible enough to keep up with technological innovation while also providing strong protection for health data."

The future of data protection laws in healthcare will likely see greater international collaboration and the adoption of best practices to address emerging challenges.

General Data Protection Regulation (GDPR)

This is European Union legislation that came into force in May 2018. Its main objective is to strengthen and unify the protection of the personal data of EU citizens and regulate the way in which organizations process this data.

Consent is a central element in the (GDPR). In short, that is, it is a free, specific, informed and unequivocal manifestation of the interested party's will, through which he or she accepts, by means of a declaration or unequivocal positive act, that his or her personal data are subject to treatment.

The right to portability, in turn, allows individuals to receive their personal data in a structured, commonly used and machine-readable format, and to have the right to transmit this data to another organization without obstacles, when technically possible.

Therefore, individuals have the power to transfer their data from one company to another, facilitating the exchange between service providers.

These rights aim to strengthen individuals' control over their own personal data, promoting transparency, accountability and the protection of privacy in the digital environment.

Healthcare institutions must be prepared to respond promptly to individuals' data access and portability requests, in accordance with the requirements established by the GDPR.

Another point is breach notification, which refers to the obligation of organizations to notify the relevant regulatory authorities, and in some cases the individuals themselves, when a data breach occurs that could pose a risk to rights and freedoms. of people.

Organizations must provide a detailed description of the nature of the violation, the possible consequences, and the measures being taken to address it.

Breach reporting is primarily intended to ensure that regulatory authorities and affected individuals are informed of data security incidents so that they can take appropriate steps to protect their rights and take corrective action if necessary.

There are sanctions imposed by the consequences set out by the GDPR for organizations that violate its provisions, including significant fines in cases of non-compliance with data protection rules.

Depending on the severity of the breach and the organization's response to corrective measures suggested by data protection authorities, fines can reach €20 million or up to 4% of the institution's annual global revenue. Whether for serious violations such as lack of data consent, violations of basic data processing principles, lack of transparency and failure to respond to data access or deletion requests.

For less serious violations, fines can be up to €10 million or up to 2% of the organization's annual global turnover, whichever is greater.

For example, these may include violations of administrative requirements, such as failure to maintain records of data processing, failure to carry out data protection impact assessments, or failure to notify a data breach to the competent authorities within the established deadline.

Health Insurance Portability and Accountability Act (HIPAA)

U.S. legislation enacted in 1996 that establishes standards for the privacy and security of health information, HIPAA applies to organizations, providers, plans, and companies that process health data on behalf of these entities.

Establishes clear rules about who can access protected health information (PHI), under what circumstances, and for what purposes.

HIPAA requires written authorization from patients before disclosing their health information to third parties, grants patients important rights over their medical records, and requires protection of personal identifiers to prevent misidentification of patients.

Additionally, the legislation addresses health data security, requiring technical, administrative, and physical safeguards to protect information against unauthorized access, misuse, and disclosure.

Health Insurance Portability and Accountability Act (HIPAA) penalties apply to healthcare organizations and other covered entities that violate its provisions, and vary depending on the severity of the violation and the specific circumstances of the case.

Civil penalties may be imposed by the U.S. Department of Health and Human Services (HHS) and are determined based on the severity of the violation.

They can range from $100 to $50,000 per violation, with an annual limit of $1,500,000 per violation type.

In more serious cases of intentional or gross negligence violation of HIPAA provisions, HHS may refer the case to the U.S. Department of Justice for investigation and possible criminal prosecution.

Criminal fines can result in prison sentences and significant fines for the individuals or organizations responsible.

In addition to civil and criminal fines, HHS may impose administrative sanctions, such as resolution agreements, correction orders, and compliance monitoring to ensure that the organization corrects its practices and complies with HIPAA.

HIPAA sanctions are intended to ensure healthcare organizations' compliance with privacy and security standards set by legislation, promoting the protection of individuals' health information and the security of healthcare data generally. .

According to Appari and Johnson (2010), HIPAA is crucial because it ensures that sensitive medical information is protected from unauthorized access, while allowing the fluidity necessary to exchange information between healthcare providers to improve the quality of care.

The legislation also requires healthcare organizations to implement physical, administrative and technical safeguards to protect patients' health information, which is vital in a context of increasing digitization of medical records.

According to Rouse (2014), HIPAA not only protects patient privacy, but also promotes public trust in the digital health system.

HIPAA compliance is essential to assure patients that their health information will be treated with the utmost confidentiality and security, which is critical to the acceptance and adoption of digital health technologies.

HIPAA establishes clear requirements for responding to data breaches, helping healthcare organizations be better prepared to deal with security incidents and minimize the impacts of potential data breaches.

As examples of actual cases in which fines have been imposed, we can mention Anthem Inc., a health insurer, which agreed to pay a record fine of $16 million in 2018 after a data breach that exposed health information of 79 million people, due to security breaches and inadequate data protection practices.

Massachusetts General Hospital agreed to pay a $1 million fine in 2011 after losing the medical records of 192 patients. The breach occurred when a hospital employee left documents containing confidential medical information on a train.

Also in 2011, Cignet Health, a Maryland medical clinic, was fined $4.3 million for refusing to provide medical records to patients upon request. These are just a few examples of cases where significant fines have been issued due to HIPAA violations.

General Data Protection Law (LGPD)

The General Data Protection Law (LGPD) is a Brazilian legislation that came into force in September 2020.

Its objective is to regulate the processing of personal data by companies and organizations in Brazil, including health data, with the aim of protecting the privacy of citizens and ensuring control over their personal information.

It is strongly inspired by the European Union's GDPR and establishes clear guidelines for the use, storage and sharing of personal data.

According to Doneda and Medaglia (2019), the LGPD is fundamental because it establishes a clear regulatory framework for the collection, storage and processing of personal data, providing greater legal certainty for both data owners and companies.

This legislation requires organizations to adopt technical and administrative measures to protect personal data, which is important to guarantee the confidentiality and integrity of the information.

According to Ferreira and Almeida (2020), the LGPD not only protects people's privacy, but also promotes public trust in the use of digital technologies.

Compliance with the LGPD is essential to assure users that their data will be treated responsibly and securely, promoting greater acceptance and use of digital services.

The sanctions provided for organizations that violate its provisions include warnings, fines of up to 2% of the company's annual revenue (limited to R$ 50 million per violation) and partial or total suspension of data processing activities.

Personal Data Protection and Electronic Documents Act (PIPEDA)

The Personal Information Protection and Electronic Documents Act (PIPEDA) is Canadian legislation that governs the collection, use and disclosure of personal information by private sector companies.

Since its implementation in 2001, PIPEDA has aimed to protect people's privacy by establishing rules on the collection, use and disclosure of personal data.

Key aspects of the law include requiring explicit consent for the collection and use of personal information, limiting the use of that information for specific purposes, the right of individuals to access and correct their own data, and the obligation of organizations to ensure the security and protection of personal data.

According to Greenberg and Roos (2015), PIPEDA is essential to protect people's privacy in the context of a rapidly growing digital environment.

In addition, PIPEDA imposes the obligation to implement appropriate security measures to protect personal information against loss, theft or unauthorized access, promoting consumer confidence in electronic transactions and the digital economy.

Bennett and Raab (2018) note that PIPEDA also plays a crucial role in harmonizing data protection practices in Canada with international standards, facilitating cross-border trade and cooperation.

PIPEDA compliance helps Canadian businesses ensure their operations comply with global privacy regulations, such as the GDPR in Europe, promoting a globally consistent approach to data protection.

PIPEDA applies to organizations doing business in Canada and is overseen by the Privacy Commissioner of Canada, who has the authority to investigate complaints and impose sanctions on organizations that fail to comply with the provisions of the law.

Sanctions imposed include investigations, hearings and consent agreements conducted by the Privacy Commissioner of Canada. In cases of non-compliance, the Commissioner can issue correction orders and seek fines through the Federal Court of Canada.

Privacy Law (Australia)

The Australian Privacy Act 1988 is crucial legislation that regulates how organizations and government agencies collect, use, store and disclose personal information.

One of the main challenges facing this legislation, as discussed by Clarke (2019), is the rapid technological evolution that continually tests the limits of the law.

Clarke argues that the constant advancement of digital technologies, such as big data, artificial intelligence and the Internet of Things (IoT), requires continuous updates and adaptations of legislation to ensure that people's privacy remains effectively protected. .

Loopholes and ambiguities in the law can be exploited, putting citizens' privacy at risk. The lack of an agile response by regulators to adjust the Privacy Law to new technological realities and emerging business practices is a significant challenge that must be addressed to maintain public trust and the protection of personal data.

Challenges of the LGPD

With the advancement of technology and the increasing digitization of information around the world, the protection of personal data has become an increasingly pressing global concern. In response to this concern, several jurisdictions have enacted data protection laws to regulate the processing of personal information by organizations and ensure the privacy and security of individuals.

However, the cross-border nature of data and the diversity of data protection laws in different countries present significant challenges for businesses and governments around the world.

Harmonizing standards is a challenge for organizations operating globally due to the diversity of data protection laws in different jurisdictions. This scenario implies high costs, administrative complexity and risk of non-compliance.

To address these challenges, companies typically take a global compliance approach, implementing policies and procedures that meet the highest data protection standards across their operations.

International cooperation and the exchange of best practices are also essential to promote the harmonization and simplification of data protection laws globally.

The security of health data is a challenge in an increasingly digitized world. With the proliferation of electronic health records, connected medical devices, and telemedicine, healthcare organizations face a growing variety of cyber threats that can compromise the privacy and integrity of patient data.

To address these challenges, organizations are investing in advanced cybersecurity technologies, fostering a culture of awareness among employees, and proactively collaborating with other industry stakeholders to identify and mitigate threats in a timely manner.

Healthcare data security is not only an ethical priority but also a regulatory requirement, with important implications for patient trust and the reputation of healthcare organizations.

The adoption of new technologies, such as artificial intelligence (AI), offers exciting opportunities to advance healthcare by enabling more accurate diagnoses, personalized treatments, and better management of health data.

However, a balance must be struck between technology-driven innovation and protecting patient data privacy. Since AI relies on large volumes of data to train and improve algorithms, concerns arise about the security and confidentiality of this data.

Therefore, healthcare organizations must implement robust cybersecurity and data privacy measures, ensuring that patients have control over how their information is collected, used and shared.

In fact, it is essential that healthcare organizations comply with data protection regulations, such as the GDPR in the European Union and the LGPD in Brazil, which establish strict requirements for the processing of personal information.

This includes implementing privacy practices by design and conducting privacy impact assessments, ensuring that patient privacy is considered at every stage of the development and implementation of AI-based technologies.

By finding the right balance between innovation and privacy protection, healthcare organizations can maximize the benefits of technology while ensuring patient trust and safety.

Education and awareness about rights and responsibilities regarding health data are essential for both patients and healthcare professionals.

Patients should understand their privacy rights, including the right to access, correct, and control the use of their health information.

On the other hand, healthcare professionals should be trained in data protection and cybersecurity best practices, ensuring they are aware of relevant laws and regulations, such as HIPAA in the United States and LGPD in Brazil.

They should also understand the importance of obtaining informed consent from patients before sharing their health information and take appropriate steps to protect the confidentiality and integrity of health data.

By promoting education and awareness of both patients and healthcare professionals, we can strengthen the protection of health data and promote a culture of security and privacy in the healthcare sector.

The diversity of data protection laws in different countries presents significant challenges for companies and governments operating in multiple jurisdictions, requiring a global and collaborative approach to ensure compliance and protection of individual rights.

Security Measures and Cybersecurity Risks

Encryption is a technique used to protect the confidentiality and integrity of information, making it unreadable to any unauthorized person.

In the healthcare context, encryption plays a key role in protecting sensitive patient data, such as medical information, diagnoses, medical records, and treatment data.

As highlighted by Martín et al. (2019), the importance of encryption in healthcare lies in the need to ensure the security and privacy of patient data, protecting it against unauthorized access, security breaches and misuse.

By encrypting this information, healthcare institutions can significantly reduce the risk of exposure to hackers and cyberattacks, ensuring data remains confidential and protected.

Access control is a crucial security measure in the context of healthcare, which aims to regulate and monitor access to health information, allowing only authorized personnel to view, modify or share sensitive patient data.

According to Schreiber et al. (2016), access control plays a critical role in protecting the confidentiality and privacy of health information, ensuring that only authorized healthcare professionals can access patients' medical records.

This measure helps mitigate the risk of security breaches and unauthorized access by protecting data from misuse or unauthorized disclosure.

Access control allows healthcare institutions to implement stronger security policies and comply with data privacy regulations such as HIPAA in the United States and GDPR in the European Union, promoting patient trust and maintaining the integrity of data. Medical records.

Malware and ransomware are types of malicious software designed to damage, access or illegally control devices, information systems or computer networks.

Malware is a general term that covers a wide variety of malicious programs, including viruses, worms, Trojan horses, and spyware, that can be used to steal sensitive information, damage systems, or perform other harmful activities.

On the other hand, ransomware is a specific type of malware that encrypts system files or blocks access to devices and demands a ransom payment to restore access or decrypt files.

According to Check Point Software Technologies Ltd., a leading cybersecurity company, malware is "harmful software code designed to cause damage to a computer, server, or network."

This malware can be distributed in various ways, such as phishing emails, infected websites, file downloads, or compromised USB devices.

Similarly, ransomware is described as "a type of malware that encrypts files on a computer system or mobile device and demands a ransom from the user to unlock access to the data."

This definition highlights the extortionist nature of ransomware, which aims to force victims to pay a ransom to regain access to their data.

The aforementioned threats pose serious information security risks and can cause significant damage to businesses and individuals, highlighting the importance of protecting against malware and ransomware through robust cybersecurity measures.

Phishing is a technique used by cybercriminals to trick people into obtaining sensitive information such as passwords, financial information or personally identifiable details.

This is usually done through emails, text messages, phone calls, or fraudulent websites posing as legitimate entities, such as banks, companies, or healthcare institutions.

Scammers often trick victims into clicking on malicious links, sharing their personal information, or downloading infected files, thereby compromising the security of their data.

In the healthcare sector, phishing can target patients, healthcare professionals, and employees of medical institutions.

For example, criminals can send spoofed emails that look like official communications from hospitals or health insurers, requesting sensitive patient information such as Social Security numbers, dates of birth, or payment information.

In fact, fraudsters can use phishing techniques to access electronic medical records systems or hospital networks, seeking to steal sensitive data or cause disruptions to healthcare services.

Phishing in healthcare can have serious consequences, including compromising patient privacy, stealing sensitive medical information, unauthorized access to healthcare systems, and disruption of medical services.

Therefore, it is essential that healthcare organizations and professionals are aware of these threats and implement robust cybersecurity measures, such as security awareness training, phishing detection systems, and data protection policies, to protect against attacks. phishing and ensuring the security of health information.

Software flaws refer to bugs, programming errors, or vulnerabilities in digital health systems and applications that can be exploited by cyber attackers to access sensitive information or compromise the integrity and availability of data.

These failures can arise for a variety of reasons, including coding errors, lack of security updates, poor software designs, or failure to implement proper security protocols.

The aforementioned vulnerabilities can be exploited in various ways, such as SQL injection attacks, denial of service (DDoS) attacks, open port exploitation, or authentication flaws.

Once attackers identify and exploit these flaws, they can gain unauthorized access to healthcare systems, electronic medical records, Internet of Things (IoT)-connected medical devices, or other sensitive medical information.

The consequences of software failures in digital health can be serious, including leakage of personal medical information, disruption of healthcare services, compromised integrity of medical records, damage to the reputation of institutions of health care and even risks to patient safety.

Therefore, it is critical that healthcare software developers adopt strong secure development practices, conduct rigorous security testing, and implement appropriate cyber protection measures to mitigate these vulnerabilities and protect the privacy and security of healthcare data.

Healthcare cyber risk mitigation strategies refer to proactive measures taken by healthcare organizations to reduce the likelihood and impact of cyber attacks on their information technology (IT) systems and infrastructure.

These strategies include a variety of technical, organizational, and governance approaches designed to protect sensitive healthcare data and ensure the security and confidentiality of patient information.

One of the key strategies is to implement strong cybersecurity measures, such as firewalls, intrusion detection systems, data encryption, multi-factor authentication, and regular software updates to fix known vulnerabilities.

Additionally, healthcare organizations should conduct regular risk assessments to identify potential threats and vulnerabilities in their systems and networks, as well as develop incident response plans to address cyberattacks in a timely manner.

Another important strategy is cybersecurity awareness and training for employees and healthcare professionals, with the goal of educating them on security best practices, threat recognition, and how to report security incidents.

This includes promoting an organizational cybersecurity culture in which all employees understand the importance of protecting health data and are committed to preventing security breaches.

According to authors Eric D. Perakslis and Kevin Fu, in their article "The Value of Security in Healthcare," "Cybersecurity in healthcare is not a technical problem, but a patient safety problem."

They highlight the importance of addressing cybersecurity challenges in healthcare as a patient safety issue, recognizing that the integrity and availability of healthcare data are critical to providing safe and effective care.

Therefore, cyber risk mitigation strategies in healthcare must be aimed at protecting the security, privacy and confidentiality of patient information, ensuring that healthcare systems and devices are resilient to cyber threats.

Startups and Medtech in Medicine

Medical technology startups and companies, known as medtechs, play a fundamental role in the innovation and transformation of the healthcare sector.

Through innovative technological solutions, these companies seek to improve the diagnosis, treatment and management of diseases, in addition to promoting more accessible and effective care for patients.

Their agility and focus on adopting new technologies have driven significant advances in medicine, offering promises of a healthier, more connected future.

A startup is an emerging company that seeks to develop an innovative and scalable business model, generally operating in an environment of uncertainty and risk.

Eric Ries, author of the book "The Lean Startup", defines a startup as "a human institution designed to create a new product or service under conditions of extreme uncertainty."

These companies often start with limited resources but seek rapid, sustainable growth through experimentation, rapid adaptation, and continuous pursuit of market opportunities.

The main goal of a startup is to find a product or service that meets market needs in a unique and effective way, often challenging established norms and introducing disruptive innovations.

In recent years, the field of medicine has witnessed a significant transformation driven by technological innovation.

Startups are playing an increasingly important role in the transformation of medicine, working in various areas to drive innovation and improve healthcare.

One such area is digital health, where startups develop mobile apps, online platforms, and connected devices to make it easier for patients to access medical information, monitor health, and manage chronic diseases.

These solutions offer greater convenience and autonomy to patients while providing healthcare professionals with real-time data.

In fact, startups are revolutionizing telemedicine, offering virtual doctor consultation services that eliminate geographic barriers and improve access to healthcare, especially in remote areas.

Another field of activity for startups in medicine is artificial intelligence (AI) and data analysis, where advanced algorithms are used to interpret large volumes of medical information and generate useful information for diagnoses, prognoses and treatments.

These solutions are applied in areas such as radiology, pathology, genomics and precision medicine, helping healthcare professionals make more precise and personalized decisions.

Some focus on improving the efficiency and quality of healthcare systems, developing solutions for electronic medical records management, optimizing hospital processes, logistics of medications and medical supplies, and patient engagement.

These initiatives aim to reduce operating costs, improve care coordination and increase patient satisfaction, contributing to the construction of more sustainable and patient-centered health systems.

Unlike traditional healthcare structures, startups have the ability to experiment and iterate quickly, accelerating the pace of progress in medicine.

As a consequence, it leads to the emergence of new therapies, advanced medical devices and more effective treatment approaches, which directly benefit patients with more modern and efficient care options.

Another important benefit of startups in medicine is the personalization and adaptation of healthcare solutions to the specific needs of patients.

Using technologies such as artificial intelligence and data analytics, these companies can develop highly personalized therapies and interventions, taking into account each individual's genetic, environmental and lifestyle factors.

Therefore, medical startups play a crucial role in promoting environmental sustainability in the healthcare sector. Through innovation in materials, production technologies and sustainable business practices, these companies are reducing the environmental impact of the healthcare industry by minimizing waste, emissions and consumption of natural resources.

In this scenario, many medical startups face challenges related to acceptance and adoption by healthcare professionals and patients.

There is often resistance to change from doctors and other healthcare providers, who may be reluctant to adopt new technologies or treatment approaches.

Lack of awareness about the benefits of solutions developed by startups and the need for additional training can also be obstacles to their adoption.

Finally, medical startups face financial sustainability and business model challenges. Many of these companies operate in a highly competitive environment where rapid innovation and scalability are essential for success.

To remain active, these innovative companies have joined technological hubs with universities, hospitals, manufacturers, laboratories, among other actors in the health industry.

Medtech, short for "medical technology" in English, refers to the use of technology to develop innovative and advanced solutions in the field of health.

Although there is no specific definition of "medical technology" by a particular author, the term is widely recognized in industry and literature as a combination of medicine and technology.

These technologies may include medical devices, diagnostic equipment, medical software, mobile applications and other innovations that aim to improve healthcare delivery, diagnosis, treatment and monitoring of patients.

These companies are at the forefront of adopting emerging technologies such as artificial intelligence, big data analytics, and advanced medical devices.

By integrating these technologies into medical solutions, medical technologies can significantly improve the diagnosis, treatment and management of diseases, providing more precise and personalized assistance to patients.

Medical technologies are often more agile and flexible compared to traditional healthcare institutions, allowing them to develop and implement innovative solutions more quickly and efficiently.

This skill is especially valuable in a constantly evolving healthcare environment, where the ability to quickly adapt to change is essential.

By collaborating with healthcare professionals and other stakeholders, medical technologies can create customized solutions that address specific needs and provide tangible benefits for patients, physicians, and healthcare institutions.

Data Interoperability in Healthcare

Healthcare data interoperability is a crucial area involving the ability of healthcare systems to share and use information effectively and securely across different platforms and organizations.

According to Kern et al. (2016), data interoperability in healthcare can be defined as "the ability of different healthcare systems and organizations to work together to use health information effectively across the healthcare sphere."

On the other hand, HIMSS (Healthcare Information and Management Systems Society) defines data interoperability as "the ability of healthcare systems to work together, within and between organizations, sharing healthcare information in an accurate, consistent and useful way."

This definition emphasizes the importance of accuracy, consistency, and usefulness of shared information, highlighting that interoperability is not just limited to the exchange of data, but also the ability to use that information in a meaningful way to support decision making. clinical and operational.

Interoperability in health encompasses different levels, each of which represents a specific degree of complexity in the exchange of information between systems.

The first level, called basic interoperability, is essential to establish communication between different systems, allowing the transfer of data, although it does not guarantee its interpretation or proper use.

Next comes syntactic interoperability, where systems not only communicate but also exchange data in standard formats and structures, making it easier to understand and integrate incoming data.

Finally, semantic interoperability allows not only structured exchange, but also the interpretation of the meaning of the exchanged data, using controlled vocabularies and standardized ontologies to ensure consistent interpretation.

These levels are essential to building an integrated and efficient digital health infrastructure.

As healthcare organizations move from basic to syntactic and finally semantic interoperability, they can ensure that data is exchanged effectively, understood correctly, and used in accordance with regulations, resulting in a better quality of care and operational efficiency.

Organizational interoperability also plays an important role, coordinating and integrating business processes and policies between different healthcare entities to ensure effective and secure collaboration in data sharing.

In summary, levels of interoperability, from basic to semantic, are essential to building an integrated health system.

Each level represents a step in the development of a digital infrastructure that facilitates the exchange of information between health systems, promoting accurate diagnoses, personalized treatments and more efficient and economical operations.

Therefore, organizational interoperability complements these levels, ensuring that data exchange occurs securely and in compliance with regulations, promoting effective collaboration between healthcare entities.

By moving from basic to syntactic and semantic interoperability, and finally to organizational interoperability, healthcare organizations can ensure that data is exchanged effectively, understood correctly, and used securely and in accordance with regulations. regulations, resulting in better quality of care and operational efficiency.

There are a number of important benefits for both healthcare professionals and patients. First, interoperability allows professionals to have access to complete and up-to-date patient information, facilitating more accurate diagnoses and personalized treatments.

It occurs because there is a guarantee that relevant data is available when needed, reducing the likelihood of medical errors resulting from incomplete or misinterpreted information.

By eliminating redundancies and simplifying administrative processes, interoperability promotes more efficient and cost-effective operation within healthcare systems, freeing up time and resources that can be spent on improving patient care.

For patients, data interoperability results in better continuity of care. With efficient information sharing between different healthcare providers, there is less need to repeat exams and procedures, ensuring a more seamless and integrated experience.

Implementing interoperability in healthcare faces a number of complex challenges that must be overcome to ensure its success.

One of the main obstacles is the incompatibility of data standards between different systems, which makes efficient integration and information sharing difficult.

This disparity in formats and structures can generate difficulties in the interpretation and use of data, compromising the effectiveness of the system as a whole.

Sharing sensitive data, such as patient health information, also requires strict security measures and compliance with privacy regulations such as GDPR in Europe and HIPAA in the United States.

Adapting legacy systems and implementing new technologies also presents challenges, as this can require substantial investments in financial and technical resources.

The complexity of updating existing systems and integrating new technology solutions can be a significant barrier for many healthcare organizations. It requires close collaboration between multiple stakeholders, including healthcare providers, technology developers, regulators and patients.

Coordinating these efforts and aligning interests often requires a strategic and multifaceted approach, further increasing the complexity of the implementation process.

There are several interoperability initiatives and standards that play a key role in promoting the effective exchange of health data between systems and organizations. One of these initiatives is FHIR (Fast Healthcare Interoperability Resources), developed by HL7, which establishes a standard for the exchange of electronic health data.

FHIR facilitates the integration of healthcare systems by defining a common framework for information exchange, thus promoting greater interoperability between different platforms and applications.

Another important initiative is IHE (Integrating the Healthcare Enterprise), which promotes the interoperability of health IT systems.

IHE defines integration profiles that guide the implementation of standards, facilitating the integration of health systems and ensuring more efficient and accurate data exchange.

Organizations such as the ONC (Office of the National Coordinator for Health Information Technology) in the US and the EU eHealth Network in Europe play an important role in developing policies and programs to promote interoperability and ensure Compliance with data security and privacy regulations.

These initiatives and standards are essential to drive collaboration between healthcare systems and facilitate more effective and secure information exchange for the benefit of patients and healthcare professionals.

Data sharing in the healthcare sector is essential to creating a more efficient, secure and patient-centered healthcare system. While there are significant implementation challenges, the potential benefits make interoperability an essential goal for healthcare organizations around the world.

Command Center

Data interoperability in healthcare is essential to improve the effectiveness of command centers, control centers that coordinate operations in healthcare institutions.

It allows the integration of systems and devices, facilitating the exchange of information in real time between different areas, which improves operational efficiency, care coordination and emergency response, by allowing more data-based decision making.

The "command center", also known as a control room, is a centralized environment equipped with advanced technology and monitoring tools, designed to monitor and manage real-time operations in various sectors, such as security, transportation, healthcare and emergencies.

Smith et al. (2016) emphasizes that these centers offer a comprehensive and integrated vision of ongoing activities, allowing efficient coordination and a rapid response to critical events or situations.

According to Jones (2018), "command centers" are typically equipped with camera monitoring systems, interactive control panels, video screens, and data analysis software to track and analyze information in real time.

These technologies allow operators to monitor ongoing events, quickly identify emerging issues or trends, and make informed decisions to optimize operational performance.

For Brown (2020), "command centers" also serve as communication and coordination centers, allowing collaboration between different teams and departments.

Through integrated communications systems, operators can communicate instantly, share relevant information and coordinate effective responses to emergency or unforeseen situations.

Therefore, "command centers" play a fundamental role in the efficient management and coordination of complex operations in different sectors, providing an integrated, rapid and informed view of ongoing activities.

The implementation of command centers in the healthcare field represents a significant advance in the management and operation of healthcare services.

Inspired by command centers used in industries such as aviation and the military, these high-tech centers are designed to monitor, coordinate and optimize hospital operations in real time.

The main objective is to improve efficiency, patient safety and quality of care.

A Command Center in the healthcare sector is a fundamental infrastructure for the effective and coordinated management of various operations within a medical institution.

Its features include real-time monitoring of key indicators, such as bed availability, patient flow and the use of medical resources.

This continuous monitoring capability enables rapid response to emergency events and optimization of operational processes to ensure efficient, quality patient care.

More than monitoring, a healthcare Command Center also plays a crucial role in data analysis. Using advanced analytics and artificial intelligence tools, it is possible to process large volumes of clinical and operational data to identify relevant patterns, trends and insights.

This analytical capability informs strategic decision making, enabling more proactive and evidence-based management.

Resource coordination is another essential functionality of a healthcare Command Center. Through integrated systems, Command Center facilitates the efficient allocation of medical personnel, equipment, medications and other resources, ensuring they are available when and where they are needed most. This optimizes the workflow and minimizes the overload of resources in certain areas of the institution.

By managing beds and patient flow, you monitor occupancy and identify opportunities for optimization, helping to reduce wait times. As a consequence, it impacts a more fluid and satisfactory experience for patients, in addition to contributing to the operational efficiency of the institution.

Another point is to facilitate communication and collaboration by providing a centralized platform for information exchange between medical, administrative and support teams.

This integrated, real-time communication is essential for a coordinated response to emergency situations and informed decision making at all levels of the healthcare institution.

Therefore, the benefits of a Health Command Center are diverse and positively impact both the internal management of medical institutions and the quality of care provided to patients.

First, the implementation of a Command Center provides a comprehensive, real-time view of hospital operations, allowing for more agile and informed decision-making.

By monitoring key indicators, such as bed occupancy, patient flow and resource availability, the Command Center allows managers to quickly identify areas of congestion, bottlenecks or emergency needs, enabling the implementation of solutions. immediate measures to optimize hospital operations.

By processing large volumes of clinical and operational information, Command Center provides valuable information to improve internal processes, allocate resources more efficiently, and anticipate future demands.

Implementing a Command Center in the healthcare sector also faces a number of challenges and important considerations that must be taken into account. First, integrating heterogeneous systems and data sources can be a major obstacle.

Cultural and organizational change is a crucial aspect to consider. The introduction of a Command Center requires a change in the mindset and work practices of medical and administrative teams.

It is essential to engage and train healthcare professionals so that they understand the value of the Command Center and are willing to adopt new processes and technologies.

This requires an ongoing training and communication effort to ensure buy-in and collaboration from all involved.

Another challenge is ensuring the reliability and accuracy of the data used by the Command Center. Data quality is essential for assertive and effective decision making.

Quality assurance and data governance mechanisms need to be implemented to ensure that the information analyzed is accurate, up-to-date and complete.

The requirements are to standardize data collection processes, implement verification and validation protocols, and define clear responsibilities to maintain data quality.

It is essential to ensure that Command Center complies with data protection regulations, such as GDPR in Europe and HIPAA in the United States, and that appropriate cybersecurity measures are implemented to protect data from unauthorized access or breaches.

The financial investment and resources required to implement and maintain a Command Center are aspects that cannot be underestimated. The construction and operation of a

Command Center requires significant investments in technological infrastructure, specialized software, qualified personnel and training.

Therefore, it is essential to conduct a careful return on investment analysis and ensure that the potential benefits justify the costs associated with implementing Command Center in healthcare.

Some hospitals and health systems around the world have already successfully implemented command centers. Johns Hopkins, one of the pioneers, uses a command center to monitor and optimize its bed capacity, significantly reducing wait times and improving patient flow efficiency.

The Hospital das Clínicas of the Faculty of Medicine of the University of São Paulo (HCFMUSP) implemented a

While Command Centers in the healthcare sector represent an exciting evolution in the healthcare landscape, it is essential to carefully address the associated challenges and considerations to maximize their potential and ensure they contribute significantly to the continuous improvement of healthcare service delivery.

Open Health

Data interoperability in healthcare is a requirement to achieve the vision of data being accessible, secure and used ethically to improve health outcomes.

This leads to broader, more integrated collaboration, driving innovation, research and the delivery of patient-centered care.

According to a study by García-Gómez et al. (2019), Open Health is defined as a model in which health data is shared openly and transparently between patients, healthcare professionals and other stakeholders, promoting collaboration and innovation in healthcare delivery.

Smith and Jones (2020) expand this definition, highlighting that Open Health is not limited only to clinical data, but also encompasses information on lifestyle, genetics, and other aspects relevant to health.

Johnson et al. (2021) emphasize that Open Health goes beyond simply sharing data, incorporating governance, ethics and security principles to ensure that the benefits of this approach are achieved without compromising the privacy and confidentiality of patient information.

These authors converge on the idea that Open Health has the potential to radically transform the way healthcare is delivered and managed, empowering patients, promoting innovation, and improving health outcomes.

The concept of Open Health represents a movement towards transparency, interoperability and data sharing in the healthcare sector.

The central idea is that health data is accessible, usable and shareable between different systems and stakeholders, including health professionals, patients, researchers and technology developers.

Open Health seeks to promote a culture of collaboration and innovation, improving the quality of care, the efficiency of health services and the empowerment of patients.

It is based on essential principles that guide its operation and mission. Transparency is one of those principles and is crucial when it comes to health data.

The information must be transparent and accessible to everyone involved, from patients and healthcare professionals to researchers, guaranteeing safe and ethical access to it.

This access not only strengthens trust in the health system, but also facilitates effective collaboration and informed decision-making at all levels.

Transparency of health data is an essential basis for ensuring quality health care and continuously promoting research and innovation in the health sector.

Interoperability is another fundamental principle of Open Health. It is essential to ensure that different healthcare systems can exchange and interpret data efficiently and accurately.

When healthcare systems are interoperable, data can flow freely between them, offering a complete and accurate view of a patient's medical history.

This interoperability not only improves care coordination, but also promotes more informed and effective decision making by healthcare professionals. It is a vital element to ensure high-quality, integrated healthcare at all levels of the healthcare system.

Open Health actively promotes collaboration between a wide range of stakeholders, including governments, healthcare institutions, technology companies and patient organizations.

Collaboration is essential to drive innovation, improve healthcare, and address complex healthcare challenges more effectively.

By joining forces, stakeholders can share knowledge, resources and experiences, developing more comprehensive and holistic solutions to health problems.

It also facilitates the exchange of information and best practices, promoting a more integrated and patient-centered approach to healthcare delivery. Ultimately, collaboration is key to creating a more efficient, accessible and wellness-oriented healthcare system for all.

Patient empowerment is another core principle of Open Health. The concept advocates that patients should have access to their own health data and be empowered to use it to make informed decisions about their own care.

Therefore, patients must have control and autonomy over their medical information, being able to access it in an easy and understandable way.

By having access to their health data, patients can become active partners in the care process, better understanding their condition, medical history, and treatment options. This access not only strengthens the relationship between patients and healthcare professionals, but also allows patients to actively participate in decisions related to their health and well-being.

Therefore, patient empowerment is essential to promote a patient-centered approach in healthcare delivery and improve clinical outcomes and patient satisfaction.

Innovation is a crucial pillar of Open Health. It recognizes that open access to health data is a key catalyst for the development of new technologies, treatments and methods of care.

By making health data accessible and ethical, Open Health fosters collaboration and creativity across the healthcare ecosystem.

Therefore, it enables researchers, healthcare professionals, technology companies and other stakeholders to use this data to identify trends, discover insights and develop innovative solutions to healthcare challenges.

Open access to healthcare data can lead to significant advances in areas such as personalized medicine, early disease diagnosis, remote patient monitoring, and more.

Adopting the Open Health concept brings with it a number of important benefits that promote a more transparent, collaborative and patient-centered approach to healthcare delivery.

From improvements in quality of care and operational efficiency to patient empowerment and advances in research and innovation.

By enabling open and secure access to healthcare data, Open Health drives positive transformation across the healthcare ecosystem, leading to better outcomes for patients and healthcare professionals.

Easy and quick access to complete and accurate data enables healthcare professionals to make more informed decisions and provide high-quality care. Interoperable systems reduce redundancy, minimize errors, and improve coordination between different healthcare providers.

Despite the significant benefits that Open Health offers, its implementation faces a number of considerable challenges. These obstacles can range from technical issues to challenges related to security and cultural acceptance.

Let's explore these challenges to better understand the complex aspects involved in the successful adoption and implementation of Open Health.

Ensuring the protection of health data from unauthorized access and privacy violations is of utmost importance. It requires implementing strong cybersecurity measures and strict compliance with privacy regulations.

The lack of unified standards can pose a significant challenge to the exchange and interpretation of data between different systems. Therefore, the adoption of common standards, such as FHIR (Fast Healthcare Interoperability Resources), becomes essential to facilitate this interoperability.

The transition to an Open Health system may require substantial investments in technology and infrastructure. Establishing clear policies and governance structures for data sharing is essential to ensure the ethical and responsible use of health data.

Several countries and organizations are successfully implementing Open Health initiatives. In the United States, the Medicare Blue Button program allows beneficiaries to download and share their health data.

The ONC (Office of the National Coordinator of Health Information Technologies) initiative promotes interoperability and the use of open standards.

The eHealth Network in Europe project works to create a European health data space, facilitating the secure exchange of health data between member countries.

In Brazil, the SUS (Sistema Único de Saúde) is developing initiatives to digitize and share health data in a secure and accessible way, including the use of electronic medical records.

Open Health therefore has the potential to significantly transform the healthcare sector by promoting greater transparency, collaboration and innovation.

While there are challenges to overcome, the potential benefits in terms of quality of care, operational efficiency, patient empowerment and research advancements are enormous.

With a coordinated effort between governments, healthcare institutions, technology companies and patients, Open Health can lead to a more integrated, effective and patient-centered healthcare system.

Health Ecosystems

The efficient and secure exchange of clinical information and medical records facilitates the development of integrated healthcare ecosystems and promotes Open Health initiatives, driving innovation and the delivery of personalized, patient-centered care.

The term "Health Ecosystems" has been addressed by different authors, offering diverse perspectives on its meaning and implications.

According to Greenwood and Dobson (2018), health ecosystems are defined as complex networks of interactions between the various actors and elements that influence the health of a population, including health institutions, professionals, patients, government and private organizations, and even socioeconomic and environmental. factors.

This definition highlights the interconnected and dynamic nature of health systems, emphasizing the importance of a holistic approach to understanding and addressing health challenges.

On the other hand, Sturmberg and Martin (2020) expand this definition, describing health ecosystems as complex adaptive systems that self-organize in response to environmental demands and changes.

They highlight the need to recognize and value the diversity and heterogeneity of actors and elements within these ecosystems, and advocate for a more flexible and adaptive approach to managing and improving health.

There is a view that health ecosystems are characterized by their complexity and dynamism, and that a deeper understanding of these systems is essential to promote effective and sustainable health interventions.

The concept of healthcare ecosystem refers to an integrated set of organizations, technologies and individuals that interact and collaborate to provide healthcare.

These ecosystems are characterized by their complexity and interdependence, where each part plays a crucial role in promoting the health and well-being of patients.

Creating effective healthcare ecosystems is critical to addressing modern healthcare challenges, such as growing demand for services, aging populations, and the need for continuous innovation.

A healthcare ecosystem is made up of a series of interconnected elements that collaborate to provide quality healthcare and promote patient well-being.

At the center are the patients themselves, who are the main beneficiaries of health services. Increasingly active and informed, patients play a crucial role in managing their own health and in the healthcare decision-making process.

Healthcare professionals, including doctors, nurses, pharmacists and other direct care providers, are key players in the functioning of the ecosystem.

Their skills and experience are essential to diagnose, treat and prevent diseases, providing personalized and effective care to patients. Healthcare institutions, such as hospitals, clinics, laboratories and other healthcare facilities, constitute the physical pillars of the ecosystem and provide the environment and resources necessary for the delivery of healthcare.

Health information technology (HIT) plays an increasingly important role, providing electronic health record systems, mobile health applications, telemedicine, and other tools that facilitate communication, data sharing, and more efficient and efficient care delivery. integrated.

The Pharmaceutical and Medical Device Industry contributes to the ecosystem by developing medicines, vaccines, medical equipment and diagnostic technologies that help prevent, diagnose and treat diseases.

Payers and insurers play a crucial role in financing healthcare, providing public and private health insurance that enables access to necessary medical services.

Regulators and governments establish policies, regulations and guidelines to ensure the quality and safety of healthcare services, protecting patients' rights and promoting equity in access to healthcare.

Finally, research and education organizations, such as universities, research institutes, and educational organizations, play a vital role in training new health professionals and conducting research that advances medical knowledge and drives innovation in the field. sector.

These various components work together to create a dynamic, collaborative, patient-centered healthcare environment.

The creation of an integrated healthcare ecosystem offers a series of benefits that positively impact both patients, healthcare professionals and institutions in the sector. One of the main benefits is the improvement in the quality of service.

Data integration and collaboration between different parts of the ecosystem result in more coordinated and personalized care for patients, ensuring a holistic and patient-centered approach.

Another point is the significantly improved operational efficiency. Interoperability and automation reduce redundancies and waste, improving the efficiency of healthcare services and enabling more effective allocation of resources. Innovation is also encouraged within an integrated healthcare ecosystem.

Collaboration between healthcare institutions, technology companies and research organizations accelerates the development and implementation of new technologies and treatments, leading to significant advances in healthcare delivery.

It also increases accessibility to healthcare. A well-coordinated ecosystem can expand access to care, especially through technologies such as telemedicine, which enable the delivery of remote medical services and connection with specialists in remote areas.

Finally, the financial and environmental sustainability of the health system is promoted. Operational efficiency and continuous innovation contribute to the financial sustainability of health institutions, while reducing environmental impact through the optimization of resources and processes.

We can cite the collaboration and alignment of all stakeholders as a requirement for the success of a healthcare ecosystem. Ensuring that all organizations and professionals involved are aligned in terms of goals and practices can be complex and requires effective communication and clear governance.

Regulation also represents a significant challenge, as healthcare ecosystems must navigate varied and often strict regulations.

This requires a thorough understanding of applicable laws and regulations and the development of appropriate compliance strategies.

Implementing new technologies and processes often requires a cultural change and ongoing training to ensure that everyone involved is prepared to adopt and effectively use the new tools and practices.

By addressing these challenges proactively and collaboratively, healthcare ecosystems can overcome obstacles and reach their full potential to improve healthcare.

Several countries and regions are successfully developing integrated healthcare ecosystems, promoting collaboration between different stakeholders and driving improvements in healthcare.

In the United States, the healthcare ecosystem is characterized by a vast network of hospitals, insurance providers, technology companies, and regulatory agencies.

Initiatives such as the Health Information Exchange (HIE) have been implemented to promote interoperability and facilitate the exchange of data between the different components of the health system.

In the European Union, the European Health Data Space project aims to create a unified digital environment for the exchange of health data between member countries. This initiative aims to improve cross-border research and care by promoting closer and more effective collaboration between European health systems.

Singapore is another example of a country with a highly integrated and efficient healthcare ecosystem. Singapore's healthcare system is known for its integration and efficient use of technology, with a clear focus on coordinated, patient-centered care.

The adoption of innovative technologies and emphasis on collaboration between different stakeholders have been critical to the success of Singapore's healthcare system.

These examples demonstrate how building integrated healthcare ecosystems can lead to significant improvements in healthcare and the patient experience, promoting a more holistic and coordinated approach to healthcare delivery.

Healthcare ecosystems represent a holistic and integrated approach to healthcare delivery, where collaboration and technology play crucial roles.

Although there are significant challenges to implementing it, the potential benefits in terms of quality of care, efficiency and innovation make building effective healthcare ecosystems an essential goal for the future of the healthcare sector.

With coordinated efforts and investments in interoperability and security, healthcare ecosystems can transform the way healthcare is delivered, benefiting patients and healthcare professionals around the world.

Digital Maturity in Healthcare Institutions

Digital maturity in healthcare refers to the level of development and capacity of a healthcare organization to effectively use digital technologies to improve its processes, services and clinical outcomes.

According to HIMSS (Healthcare Information and Management Systems Society), digital maturity can be defined as "a healthcare organization's ability to assess, plan, and implement effective digital strategies to improve quality of care, patient safety, and operating efficiency".

It involves not only the adoption of digital technologies, but also the integration and optimization of these technologies in all aspects of healthcare delivery.

According to consulting firm Deloitte, digital maturity in healthcare also encompasses an organization's ability to intelligently and strategically use data to inform clinical and operational decisions.

It includes the collection, analysis and interpretation of clinical, administrative and financial data to identify patterns, trends and opportunities for improvement.

In summary, digital maturity in healthcare is not just limited to the adoption of technologies, but also encompasses the ability to use these technologies in an effective, data-driven manner to generate better outcomes for patients and the organization as a whole. .

HIMSS (Health Information and Management Systems Society) offers two digital maturity assessment models widely recognized in the healthcare sector: the EMRAM (Electronic Medical Records Adoption Model) and the O-EMRAM (Electronic Medical Records Adoption Model). for Outpatients).

These models provide a framework for evaluating the stage of adoption and utilization of electronic medical records in hospitals and outpatient clinics, respectively.

EMRAM evaluates the adoption of electronic medical records systems in hospital settings, providing a seven-stage scale ranging from simple computerization to full utilization of electronic medical records.

Each stage represents a progressively higher level of integration and utilization of technology to improve healthcare and operational efficiency.

On the other hand, O-EMRAM is specific for outpatient settings, such as doctors' offices and clinics. This model follows a similar structure to EMRAM, but adapted to evaluate the adoption of electronic medical records in outpatient settings.

Both HIMSS models provide a comprehensive assessment of digital health maturity and help organizations identify areas of opportunity for improvement and development in the area of health information technology.

Recognized for its expertise in healthcare digital maturity assessment and consulting services, Ernst & Young (EY) helps organizations assess their readiness and ability to embark on the digital transformation journey.

Using tailored approaches, EY works closely with its clients to understand their specific needs and deliver solutions that drive innovation and digital progress in healthcare.

Conclusion

As we say goodbye to this exploration of digital health and glimpse the future of healthcare, it is clear that we are witnessing an unprecedented revolution in the healthcare sector.

The intersection of technology and medicine is opening new horizons, promoting a more integrated, personalized and patient-centered approach to healthcare delivery.

One of the fundamental pillars of this advance is data exchange. As healthcare systems become increasingly interconnected and interoperable, the free flow of information between patients, healthcare professionals, medical institutions and technology companies is transforming the way we understand and approach healthcare.

Access to accurate, real-time data allows for faster and more accurate diagnoses, more effective treatments, and smoother coordination between different points of care.

The "Patient Journey" emerges as a central concept in digital health. By taking a holistic, patient-centered approach, health systems are recognizing the importance of considering not only the physical, but also the emotional, social and behavioral aspects of health.

Empowering patients to manage their own health by providing them with relevant tools and information is becoming a crucial priority in healthcare delivery.

To move into the future, it is essential that we continue to prioritize data sharing and the patient journey as cornerstones of digital health.

This will require collaboration among all stakeholders in the healthcare ecosystem, as well as continued investments in technology infrastructure, cybersecurity, and patient education.

However, as we face the challenges that accompany this transformation, we must also celebrate the opportunities it offers.

Digital health offers us the opportunity to reimagine and reinvent the healthcare system to make it more accessible, efficient and patient-centered.

With a collaborative, future-oriented approach, we can build a world where everyone has access to quality healthcare and where the patient journey is truly empowering and transformative.

Glossary of Technical Terms

EHR (Electronic Health Record): Electronic Health Record A digital system for storing patients' medical information.

Telemedicine: Provision of health services remotely through communication technologies, such as video conferencing and telephone calls.

Wearables: Portable electronic devices that monitor and record data related to the user's health and well-being.

Interoperability: the ability of different systems and devices to exchange and use information in a consistent manner.

Artificial intelligence (AI): Technology that enables computer systems to perform tasks that typically require human intelligence, such as pattern recognition, learning, and decision-making.

Big Data: An extremely large and complex set of data that can be analyzed to reveal patterns, trends, and associations.

Blockchain: Distributed, immutable ledger system that can be used to ensure data security and transparency.

GDPR (General Data Protection Regulation): European regulation that defines strict standards for the protection of personal data.

HIPAA (Health Insurance Portability and Accountability Act): US law that protects patients' medical information.

Bibliographic References

Books and academic articles.

ATZORI, L.; IERA, A.; MORABITO, G. The Internet of Things: A survey. Computer Networks, v. 54, no. 15, p. 2787-2805, 2010.

BASHSHUR, RL; SHANNON, GW; KRUPINSKI, EA The Definition of Telemedicine. Telemedicine and e-Health, v. 25, no. 3, p. 235-237, 2019.

BATES, D.W.; EBELL, M.; GOTLIEB, E.; ZAPP, J.; MULLINS, HC A proposal for electronic medical records in US primary care. Journal of the American Medical Informatics Association, v. 10, no. 1 p. 1–10, 2003. DOI: 10.1197/jamia.M1092

BATES, D.W.; LEAPE, LL; CULLEN, DJ; LAIRD, N.; PETERSEN, LA; TEICH, JM; ... SEGER, DL Effect of computerized physician order entry and a team intervention on prevention of serious medication errors. JAMA, v. 280, no. 15, p. 1311-1316, 2003.

BENNETT, C.; RAAB, C. The Harmonization of Data Protection Practices through PIPEDA. Journal of International Data Privacy Law, v. 12, no. 3, p. 115-130, 2018.

BLUMENTHAL, D. Launching HITECH. The New England Journal of Medicine, v. 364, no. 5 p. 382-385, 2011. DOI: 10.1056/NEJMp1012825

BUNTIN, MB; BURKE, MF; HOAGLIN, MC; BLUMENTHAL, D. The benefits of health information technology: A review of the recent literature shows predominantly positive results. Health Affairs, v. 30, no. 3, p. 464-471, 2011.

BUYYA, R. Internet of Things: Principles and Paradigms. Academic Press, 2018.

EYSENBACH, G. What is e-health? Journal of Medical Internet Research, v. 3, no. 2, e20, 2001.

GAGNÉ, M.; DUBUC, M. Robotic Surgery Platforms: Features and Applications. Surgical Innovations, v. 15, no. 1 p. 25-40, 2018.

GARCÍA-GÓMEZ, JM; GONZÁLEZ, R.; PÉREZ, S. Open Health: Data Sharing Models for Collaborative and Innovative Healthcare. International Journal of Medical Informatics, v. 15, no. 3, p. 220-235, 2019.

GEE, PM; PATERNITI, DA; WARD, D.; SOEDERBERG MILLER, LM e-Patients perceptions of using personal health records for self-management support of chronic illness. Computers, Informatics, Nursing, v. 33, no. 6, p. 229-237, 2015.

GUBBI, J.; BUYYA, R.; MARUSIC, S.; PALANISWAMI, M. Internet of Things (IoT): A vision, architectural elements, and future directions. Future Generation Computer Systems, v. 29, no. 7, p. 1645-1660, 2013.

HÄYRINEN, K.; SARANTO, K.; NYKÄNEN, P. Definition, structure, content, use and impacts of electronic health records: A review of the research literature. International Journal of Medical Informatics, v. 77, no. 5 p. 291-304, 2008. DOI: 10.1016/j.ijmedinf.2007.09.001

HOUSEMAN, T.; DREDZE, M. The impact of big data on healthcare: A review. Journal of Biomedical Informatics, v. 56, p. 207-215, 2015.

JACKSON, J.; BOREN, S. Wearable technology: Impact on health and wellness. Journal of Medical Systems, v. 43, no. 9, p. 308, 2019.

JONES, M. The Role of Command Centers in Modern Healthcare. Journal of Healthcare Technology, v. 9, no. 4, p. 180-195, 2018.

KAPLAN, B. How Should Health Data Be Used? Privacy, Secondary Use, and Big Data Sales. Cambridge Quarterly of Healthcare Ethics, v. 25, no. 2 P. 312-329, 2016.

KAY, M.; SANTOS, J.; TAKANE, M. mHealth: New horizons for health through mobile technologies. World Health Organization, v. 3, no. 7, p. 1-117, 2001.

KEESARA, S.; JONAS, A.; SCHULMAN, K. Covid-19 and health care's digital revolution. New England Journal of Medicine, v. 382, no. 23, e82, 2020.

KERN, L.M.; BARRON, Y.; DORAN, R.; ELDER, N. Interoperability of Health Data: Defining Effective Use in Healthcare. Journal of Health Informatics, v. 12, no. 3, p. 65-80, 2016.

KUMAR, S.; PURASWANI, S. Data Protection Laws in Healthcare: Ensuring Privacy and Confidentiality. Journal of Health Law and Ethics, v. 12, no. 1 p. 45-60, 2020.

MCKINSEY GLOBAL INSTITUTE. The Internet of Things: Mapping the value beyond the hype. McKinsey & Company, 2015.

NOSTA, J. The Fourth Industrial Revolution: Digital Health. Forbes, 2018.

PATEL, V.; ASHRAFIAN, H.; DARZI, A.; ATHANASIOU, T. Evaluating the role of mobile applications in improving health outcomes in cardiothoracic surgery. Annals of Thoracic Surgery, v. 99, no. 1 p. 200-207, 2015.

PATEL, V.; WANG, J. Wearable technology in medicine and health care: Wearables can provide real-time data and insights. Journal of Medical Internet Research, v. 22, no. 10, e20492, 2020.

PERAKSLIS, ED; FU, K. The Value of Safety in Healthcare. Journal of Cybersecurity in Healthcare, v. 4, no. 2 P. 85-100, 2021.

RIES, E. The Lean Startup: How Today's Entrepreneurs Use Continuous Innovation to Create Radically Successful Businesses. New York: Crown Business, 2011.

SHAH, R.; AMIN, S.; GOPAL, A. The Role of Robotic Systems in Enhancing Surgical Precision. Journal of Robotic Surgery, v. 10, no. 2 P. 115-130, 2021.

SMITH, J.; WILLIAMS, P.; JONES, L. Command Centers in Healthcare: Enhancing Coordination and Response. Healthcare Management Review, v. 21, no. 2 P. 145-160, 2016.

SMITH, MW; HOPKINS, DA Patient Journey Mapping in a Healthcare Setting. In: Improving Patient Experience. Springer, Cham, 2018. p. 29-43.

TOPOL, EJ Deep Medicine: How Artificial Intelligence Can Make Healthcare Human Again. Hachette UK, 2019.

TOPOL, EJ The Creative Destruction of Medicine: How the Digital Revolution Will Create Better Health Care. Basic Books, 2012.

WESTPHAL, J.D.; GULATI, R.; SHORTELL, SM Customization or conformity? An institutional and network perspective on the content and consequences of TQM adoption. Administrative Science Quarterly, v. 42, no. 2 P. 366-394, 2010.

Magazine and Newspaper Articles

Bertalán Meskó. (2017). The future of healthcare: the impact of digital health. *World Economic Forum* . Retrieved from https://www.weforum.org/agenda/2017/03/the-future-of-healthcare-the-impact-of-digital-health/

Oliver, D. (2016). Digital health: monitoring, technology and wearables. *The Guardian* . Obtained from https://www.theguardian.com/technology/2016/apr/07/digital-health-tracking-technology-wearables

Official Reports and Documents

World Health Organization. (2018). WHO Guideline: Recommendations on digital interventions for health system strengthening. Geneva: World Health Organization.

European Union. (2016). General Data Protection Regulation (GDPR). Official journal of the European Union.

US Department of Health and Human Services (1996). Health Insurance Portability and Accountability Act (HIPAA). Washington, DC: United States Government Printing Office.

Online resources and websites

Harvard Medical School. (2023). Digital health. Obtained from https://hms.harvard.edu/departments/digital-health

International Medical Informatics Association (IMIA). (2023). What is health informatics? Retrieved from https://imia-medinfo.org/wp/what-is-health-informatics/

National Institutes of Health (NIH). (2023). HealthIT. Obtained from https://www.nih.gov/health-information/health-it

Gupta, S., and Khanna, N. (2016). Redefining the patient journey in healthcare: A patient-centered approach. Journal of Healthcare Management, 61(4), 262–274.

Smith, J., Jones, M., and Doe, A. (2018). Understanding the patient journey: concepts and methodologies. Journal of Patient Experience, 5(1), 63–72.

Johnson, R., Brown, K., and Lee, S. (2020). Mapping the patient journey: A framework for understanding healthcare experiences. Journal of Patient Experience, 7(3), 276–286.

Case studies and practical examples

Telemedicine Institute of India. (2020). Implementation of a telemedicine network. *Annual Report of the Telemedicine Institute* .

Fitbit and heart health in the US (2021). Continuous health monitoring with wearable devices. *I study at Stanford University* .

Health applications in Africa. (2019). Malaria reduction through mobile technologies. *World Health Organization Report* .

Conferences and Symposiums

American Medical Informatics Association (AMIA) Annual Symposium. (2022). Proceedings on health IT and digital health.

HIMSS Global Health Conference and Expo. (2023). Innovations in digital health and technology.

Legislation and Regulation

General Law on Protection of Personal Data (LGPD), Brazil. (2018). Law No. 13,709.

Health Information Technology for Economic and Clinical Health (HITECH) Act (2009). United States Congress.

www.ingramcontent.com/pod-product-compliance
Lightning Source LLC
Chambersburg PA
CBHW050055230526
45470CB00004B/1541